War-Torn Exchanges

EDITED BY ANDREA McKENZIE

War-Torn Exchanges

The Lives and Letters of Nursing Sisters Laura Holland and Mildred Forbes

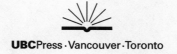

UBCPress · Vancouver · Toronto

25 24 23 22 21 20 19 18 17 16   5 4 3 2 1

Printed in Canada on FSC-certified ancient-forest-free paper
(100% post-consumer recycled) that is processed chlorine- and acid-free.

Library and Archives Canada Cataloguing in Publication

War-torn exchanges : the lives and letters of nursing sisters Laura Holland and Mildred Forbes / edited by Andrea McKenzie.

Includes bibliographical references and index.
Issued in print and electronic formats.
ISBN 978-0-7748-3254-0 (pbk.). – ISBN 978-0-7748-3255-7 (pdf). –
ISBN 978-0-7748-3256-4 (epub). – ISBN 978-0-7748-3257-1 (mobi)

1. Holland, Laura, 1883–1956 – Correspondence. 2. Forbes, Mildred, 1884–1921 – Correspondence. 3. Canada. Canadian Army Medical Corps – Nurses – Correspondence. 4. Nurses – Canada – Biography. 5. World War, 1914–1918 – Participation, Female. 6. Military nursing – Canada – History – 20th century. 7. World War, 1914–1918 – Medical care – Canada. I. Holland, Laura, 1883–1956 – Correspondence. Selections. II. Forbes, Mildred, 1884-1921 – Correspondence. Selections.

D629 C2 W37 2016   940.4'75710922   C2016-901211-5
                                                   C2016-901212-3

Canadä

UBC Press gratefully acknowledges the financial support for our publishing program of the Government of Canada (through the Canada Book Fund), the Canada Council for the Arts, and the British Columbia Arts Council.

This book has been published with the help of a grant from the Canadian Federation for the Humanities and Social Sciences, through the Awards to Scholarly Publications Program, using funds provided by the Social Sciences and Humanities Research Council of Canada.

Printed and bound in Canada by Friesens
Set in Garamond by Artegraphica Design Co. Ltd.
Copy editor: Matthew Kudelka

UBC Press
The University of British Columbia
2029 West Mall
Vancouver, BC V6T 1Z2
www.ubcpress.ca

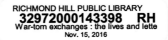

Contents

Illustrations

Acknowledgments

I would like to thank the many groups and individuals who helped to bring this work to fruition. I am grateful to the Faculty of Liberal Arts and Professional Studies at York University for funding this research in its later stages and equally grateful to Pat C. Hoy II and New York University for travel funding and support given in the initial stages of the project.

The archivists at many institutions contributed their expertise: Chris Hives and Candice Bjur at the UBC Archives; Library and Archives Canada; Susan Ross and the other helpful staff at the Canadian War Museum; the Archives of Ontario; Margaret Suttie, of the Alumnae Association of the Montreal General Hospital School of Nursing Archives; McGill University Archives; the College of Nurses of Ontario Archives; the College of Registered Nurses of British Columbia Archives; Lorraine Mychajlunow at the College and Association of Registered Nurses of Alberta Archives; and Trent University Archives.

Stephen Cooke, representing Laura Holland's family, generously shared family artifacts and photographs with me, introduced me to Laura's colleague Patricia Fulton, and conducted an interview with Patricia. With his partner, Robert Pestes, Stephen showed me Laura's Vancouver. I am exceptionally grateful to Stephen and his family. Glennis Zilm, nurse-historian, opened her home and her knowledge of Laura's postwar influence. Margaret Suttie generously contributed research about and photographs of Laura and Mildred, plus genealogical research. John Gass kindly supplied a photograph of Casualty Clearing Station No. 2 from Clare Gass's personal album. Sara Menuck and Anastasiya Ivanova gave excellent research support during this project. My sister, Allison Cline-Dean, expert genealogist, researched the Holland, Hadrill, Forbes, and Galt families and provided support throughout the project. Cynthia Toman provided encouragement and information in the later stages of the work, and Mélanie Morin-Pelletier helpfully contributed knowledge of Laura's and Mildred's immediate postwar work. I would also like to thank Carol Acton for her help in developing my ideas about women, nursing, and war over many years, and for her constant encouragement.

I could not have completed this book without Emily Andrew, editor at UBC Press, who helped me expand and refine my ideas from the proposal through to the finished book, and Lesley Erickson, production editor at UBC Press, whose expertise guided me through to the end.

Finally, my mother and family have shown exemplary patience with my disappearances into a past era, while Ro Sheffe, partner extraordinaire, has contributed in innumerable ways to this book and to my life, reading, commenting, and encouraging at every stage along the way, and researching and drawing the original maps of the Mediterranean Front and the Western Front.

Abbreviations

ANZAC	Australian and New Zealand Army Corps
CAMC	Canadian Army Medical Corps
CBE	Commander of the British Empire
CCS	Casualty Clearing Station
CSH	Canadian Stationary Hospital
CGH	Canadian General Hospital
GOC	general officer commanding
IODE	Imperial Order Daughters of the Empire
MGH	Montreal General Hospital
NCO	non-commissioned officer
NS	nursing sister
OC	officer commanding
QAIMNS	Queen Alexandra's Imperial Military Nursing Service
RAMC	Royal Army Medical Corps
RFC	Royal Flying Corps
RRC	Royal Red Cross
RTO	Railway Transport Officer

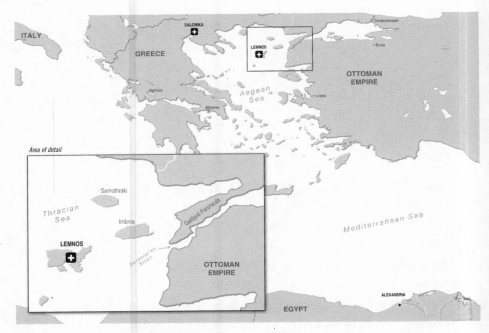

Mediterranean Front. Hospitals where Laura and Mildred nursed.

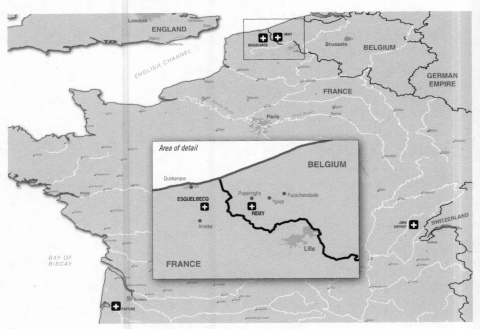

Western Front. Hospitals where Laura and Mildred nursed.

War-Torn Exchanges

Introduction:
Friendship and War

On June 4, 1915, Canadian nursing sisters Laura Holland and Mildred Forbes sailed from Montreal to Europe on their way to four tumultuous years of wartime nursing. In a letter she wrote during the voyage, Mildred promised Laura's mother, "I will always take the best care I can of Lollie [Laura] ... I would rather be torpedoed than ... separated."[1] Laura and Mildred would remain together throughout the First World War, making professional sacrifices to stay together in a relationship that was in some ways as close as a marriage. They would endure privations in what was perhaps the "worst station" of the war, the Greek island of Lemnos; be captivated by the grandeur of Cairo yet appalled at its filth and extreme poverty; explore trenches and refugees' lives in Salonika; revel in meeting royalty in London; and be shelled out of a casualty clearing station in France.[2] In May 1919, they would be discharged from the army and set sail on the same ship for Canada, still together.

The two women's wartime letters have been separated for decades – Laura's in British Columbia, Mildred's in Ottawa.[3] This book reunites their shared experiences of the war, highlighting their individual perspectives and attitudes and illuminating the friendship that sustained them both through those difficult years. Their double account of events, written by two outstanding personalities, offers a rich and compelling journey that dates from their arrival in England in 1915 to shortly before their joint discharge in 1919. Laura Holland, ARRC, CBE, LLD,[4] wrote to her widowed mother in Montreal, Laura Hadrill Holland; Mildred Forbes – RRC, Médaille des epidémies en argent, mentioned in despatches[5] – wrote to her close friend Cairine Reay

Wilson, who would one day be appointed Canada's first woman senator but who at the time was busy raising her growing family.[6] Holland and Wilson would be Canadian pioneers in the postwar world, and Holland's war experiences would influence her revolutionary work in Canadian social welfare.[7]

Narratives by nurses who served with other Allied countries have been published and are widely available.[8] First-person accounts by Canadian nurses are rare and letters rarer still. Unlike diaries and retrospective memoirs, letters home bring to light the narratives of war that nurses shared with Canadians at home. At a time when newspaper accounts were censored and when visits home by nurses were rare, letters were the primary means of communicating with family and friends. As Laura's and Mildred's letters demonstrate, despite censorship regulations, nurses' letters, with their realistic accounts of hospital life and soldiers' conditions, often undermined publicly disseminated discourses that emphasized heroism and sacrifice. Although letters by other Canadian military nurses, such as Ruby Peterkin and Luella Denton, are publicly available,[9] they are fragmented and sparse;[10] in depth and duration, only Helen Fowlds's ninety-four letters[11] compare to Mildred and Laura's joint 164 letters and approximately 200,000 words across the four years of their war.

Other historians and literary scholars have studied the correspondence between male soldiers and civilian women and found that these exchanged war stories are "defined [as much] by connectedness ... as by separation."[12] The men who fought and the women who worked at home "were not isolated, mutually indifferent communities" but were "intimately connected by networks of correspondence that kept the horrors of combat vividly present ... and the refuge of home never entirely remote."[13] For soldiers writing to their mothers, correspondence also became a means of recapturing "the lives they had left behind."[14]

Yet the letters of women on active service remain unexplored, as does the relationship between the professional nurses who worked abroad and the women who worked at home.[15] Equally lacking is an in-depth analysis of female friendships during wartime. For nurses, including the military nurses in this book, war nursing could be traumatic and draining, with friendship a primary means of sustaining equilibrium amid chaos. The letters of Laura Holland and Mildred Forbes, Canadian military nurses and best friends, enable us to explore both women's relationships and military nurses' friendships. Unlike war diaries, which were usually private, for the author's eyes only, war correspondence illuminates how the writers shaped attitudes and events for those at home, including Laura's and Mildred's views about Canadian women as active war workers. As well, unlike the diaries and letters written by a single individual, Laura and Mildred's joint correspondence reveals the role their staunch friendship played in enabling both to endure privation, illness, boredom, and emotional trauma, as well as the rich pleasure they could create even in such mundane chores as finding a new laundry for the unit. This book's objectives, then, are threefold: to study the role of friendship in Canadian military nurses' First World War lives; to explore the strategies Laura and Mildred used when representing themselves, their experiences, and the soldiers they nursed in their correspondence with Mrs. Holland and Cairine Wilson; and to make Laura's and Mildred's correspondence available to interested readers.

Laura and Mildred were two of the 2,818 trained nurses who served overseas with the Canadian Army Medical Corps (CAMC) during the First World War.[16] Alone among the Allied forces, Canadian nursing sisters held the relative rank and pay of officers and enjoyed some of the same privileges. The rank of nursing sister was equivalent to that of lieutenant, matron to that of captain, and matron-in-chief to that of major.[17] Their dress uniforms of navy-blue and their working uniforms of medium-blue with white aprons and veils carried the stars of rank – a source of pride for some but of embarrassment for others.[18] Unlike the nurses of Queen Alexandra's Imperial Military Nursing Service (QAIMNS; the QAs), who were "attached to, but not part of, the [British] Army," Canadian nurses had been an integral part of the CAMC since the Boer War.[19] Nursing in prewar Canada had become a respectable profession, with its practitioners treated accordingly, and the daughters of socially elite families (like Laura's and Mildred's) were entering its training schools. Applicants needed at least a high school education and were "expected to conform to an élite vision of sexual feminine respectability."[20] Janet S.K. Watson rightly contends that "a major shift in the status of the hospital nurse" occurred in Britain in the late nineteenth century, partly as a result of "the interest in nursing as paid employment from a new and respectable female population."[21] Yet the distinct class differences in Britain still led to "nurses ... being treated like servants" and having "no standing at all."[22]

When the Canadian nurses went overseas as part of the CAMC, they "expected British nurses to welcome them warmly and treat them as professional equals."[23] They also expected the British military administration and British citizens to treat them with respect. Yet the Canadians' position overseas was ambiguous. As female officers, they were unique, and men "of all ranks seemed to find" the Canadian nurses' authority "puzzling" because women were expected to defer to authority, not wield it.[24] Some British nurses displayed jealousy over the "officer's rank, pay, and privileges that the CAMC nurses had and the QAIMNS nurses did not."[25] Many British also considered the Canadians inferior because they were "colonials," presumably used to, as one British officer remarked, "roughing it."[26] These ambiguities and differing attitudes would make life in the military sometimes difficult to bear.

Canadian trained nurses provided essential care for ill and wounded soldiers outside the trenches. Usually, casualties received initial care at a medical post or field ambulance from a male medical team and were then transported to a casualty clearing station (CCS), whose medical staff included nurses. The turnover of patients at CCSs was rapid; soldiers were operated on and kept until their condition stabilized, or they were sent down the line to a stationary or general hospital farther away from the firing line for additional treatment. From there, men could be returned to their regiments or shipped to England for further treatment or convalescence. Hospital trains staffed with nurses and medical officers transported ill and wounded men by land;[27] hospital ships, also staffed with medical personnel, transported casualties by sea or canal. On some fronts, such as the Dardanelles, ill and wounded soldiers were treated on site, then sent by ship directly to hospitals on Imbros or Lemnos or at Alexandria, the closest locations.

Nursing work fluctuated with the fighting. Lulls in the fighting meant calm, but when an attack occurred, convoys of hundreds of men could arrive at a CCS or hospital, causing frantic work in the operating rooms and in the wards. Nurses performed vital roles, working alongside doctors to perform treatments and operations, providing essential bedside care for their physically – and often emotionally – traumatized patients, and managing administrative work to ensure the smooth flow of drugs, diets, and equipment.[28] This indispensable work was physically and emotionally draining,[29] especially given the numbers of casualties, the severity of wounds and illnesses, the shelling and bombing of some CCSs and hospitals, and the often severe climates. Throughout, the nurses maintained morale, providing comforts for their patients, flowers and treats for the wards, cheerful Christmases with decorations and special dinners, and open-house teas for male officers.[30] In all ways, their work was essential and their presence vital.

Becoming Nurses

Laura and Mildred came from similar social and cultural backgrounds; they also shared the professional ethics and discipline instilled in them during their training at the Montreal General Hospital School of Nursing. Mildred Hope Forbes was born to an elite family in Montreal on November 18, 1884, the youngest child of Matilda Torrance McPherson and Alexander Mackenzie Forbes, an insurance agent. Her mother was a descendant of the Torrances, one of Montreal's wealthiest merchant families, and her relatives included the

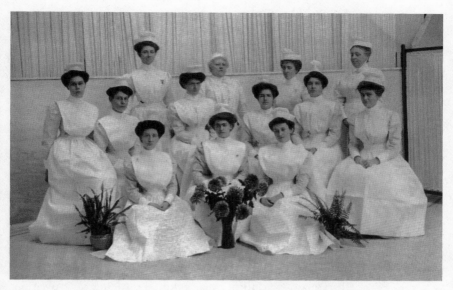

Montreal General Hospital School of Nursing class, 1908. Mildred Forbes is seated third from the right in the second row. *McGill University Archives, PL007878*

powerful Galt family. One of Mildred's half-brothers from her father's first marriage, also named Alexander Mackenzie Forbes, became a doctor and a founder of the Montreal Memorial Children's Hospital.[31] Their social circle included Canada's most influential families: the Tuppers, the Galts, Cairine Wilson's family, and others. Given this social and economic background, Mildred's decision to enter the Montreal General Hospital School of Nursing must have been from choice, perhaps influenced by her brother's medical career. She applied there and was accepted for training at the age of twenty-one in 1905, graduating in 1908. Her decision might seem unusual, but the same one was made by other daughters of prestigious families – for example, by Mildred's cousin, Cecily Galt, whose father was a judge,[32] and Juliette Pelletier,[33] who came from a well-known political family. These women, like many other Canadian women of the time, had chosen a profession that provided independence and the opportunity to lead. Studies of Canadian nurses show that women who selected nursing were from "a range of family backgrounds – middle class, working class, and agricultural."[34] The elite social status of the four nurses mentioned here speaks to the growing prestige and respectability of nursing as a profession. Given the fierce competition for overseas placement, the presence of these four in a single unit of twenty-six nurses with Canadian Stationary Hospital No. 1 speaks to their families' influence and power.

Nursing gave Mildred scope for her abilities as an administrator and organizer, as well as the freedom to travel to places such as Italy and Switzerland with a fellow nurse before the war.[35] An exceptionally able executive, she found life in the military difficult when the nursing work and the supplies were poorly organized, to the detriment of both patients and nurses – for example, on Lemnos. Her letters to Cairine Wilson are trenchant and to the point, clearly demonstrating her impatience with a supply system that did not work. For her, writing became both a means of expressing that impatience and a weapon for working outside the system to garner the supplies she and the other nurses needed to do their work effectively. Not surprisingly, her executive abilities and her social status drew the attention of Canadian matron-in-chief Margaret Macdonald.[36] As acting matron of the nurses on board the ship to England in 1915, Mildred worked closely with Miss Macdonald to place the nurses in hospitals in England and abroad. This opportunity enabled her to display her abilities – and, unconsciously, the elite social status that enabled Mildred and Laura to remain together throughout the war.

Laura Elizabeth Holland was born a year before her friend, on November 14, 1883, to Laura Elizabeth Hadrill and Arthur Hollingsworth Holland. She was the only girl in a family of four living children. Her mother was born in London, England, and in the 1870s immigrated with her parents and siblings to Montreal, where they opened a dry goods store.[37] Her father, born in Tyrconnell, Ontario, was the son of the Reverend Henry Holland, a respected clergyman who ended his long career at St. George's Anglican Church in St. Catharines, Ontario. Arthur, a commercial salesman, moved his family from Montreal to Truro, Nova Scotia, in the 1880s, then to Toronto in the late 1890s. His death in the early 1900s led his widow to return to Montreal in 1904, where her family lived with her brother George Hadrill (secretary of the Board of Trade) and his family. By the beginning of the war, Laura's mother, her uncle George, and her cousin Temple were living in adjoining apartments at 47 St. Mark Place in the affluent St-Antoine district. Temple Hadrill, born in 1895, was a cadet at the military college before he joined the Army Service Corps; he would later transfer to the Royal Flying Corps as a pilot.

Laura's route to nursing was unusual and late. She attended a private school in Toronto, studied music, then taught music for eleven years.[38] During this period, she also journeyed to Britain with her mother to visit family, visited New York City, and travelled extensively in western Canada, teaching music for a winter in Alberta.[39] Her travel diaries from that time paint a vivid picture of social life in a number of energetic western towns and cities. These two loves – music and travel – would remain with her for life, as would her need to write out her experiences. Her detailed and usually lengthy letters to her

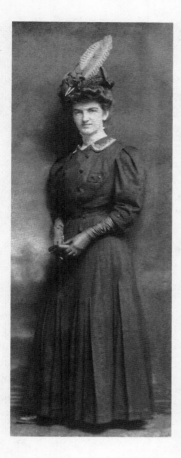

Laura ("Lollie") Holland,
circa 1907. *UBC Archives
123.1/4*

mother often took the form of diaries expanded from a daily memo book she kept. Laura's letters were a means of drawing her family into her wartime life and space, depicting her daily life and living conditions in tent and hut, the new landscapes and people she met, and the sights she saw. She spent hours writing, sometimes from her night-time ward, sometimes while Mildred was reading; some of the irritation she occasionally expressed about her fellow nurses stemmed from her need for peace to write.

We do not know when Laura and Mildred met, but it was probably between 1908 and 1910, after Laura returned from the west. Perhaps they met through church – both were Anglican – or at a social event. Perhaps it was nursing that brought them together, given that Laura entered the Montreal General Hospital School of Nursing, graduating in 1913,[40] when she was thirty years old.

By 1915, Laura and Mildred were firm friends, eager and determined to do war nursing. Given the fierce competition among nurses for overseas placements, Mildred's family connections and influence undoubtedly helped them obtain places in the same draft of nurses. They worked in a variety of medical institutions and countries during the war: at the Duchess of Connaught's Red Cross Hospital on the Astors' Cliveden estate in England; at CSH No. 1 on Lemnos and then at Salonika in 1915 and 1916; in London, where Mildred worked in Macdonald's office as her assistant in late 1916 and part of 1917, while Laura worked at No. 1 Hyde Park Place, a hospital for officers; at Crowborough, a small hospital in England that served a Canadian army camp; at CCS No. 2 at Remy Siding and Esquelbecq from mid-1917 to mid-1918, where Mildred served as acting matron; and, finally, at two small hospitals attached to Canadian Forestry Corps units in France,[41] just in time for the deadly influenza epidemic of 1918–19.

COMMUNICATING WAR

The importance of nurses' letters to Canadian First World War studies cannot be underestimated: like wartime diaries, they provide an immediacy and suspense that memoirs written in retrospect do not.[42] War correspondence is one of the only means available for us to understand just what information about events, attitudes, and personal experience reached Canadian families from the distant war in Europe and Africa. Newspaper accounts were heavily censored,[43] and personal leaves to Canada were infrequent. Nurses could visit Canada by serving on transport duty, but Laura and Mildred chose not to.[44] The pairs' letters, for the most part, ensured that their families and friends had a realistic picture of their war experiences, including the hospitals they worked in, their patients' wounds and illnesses, and their living conditions. Letters from nurses also became a way of disseminating information about the experiences of soldiers in the ranks to those at home. Hospitals and CCSs became places where different experiences of war were shared,[45] sometimes through words, and often through the physical narratives of wounds and illness, which military nurses could read and communicate to those at home. As such, nurses' letters could counteract the often romanticized or distorted public discourses surrounding nurses' and soldiers' roles and experiences during the war.

Previous studies of wartime correspondence have focused on the letters exchanged between male soldiers and female civilians and have demonstrated that dividing the "home front" from the "battle front" is an artificially imposed construction designed to privilege the experiences of male combatant soldiers.[46] What such studies have omitted is the very different setting of the war hospital, where nurses on active service disseminated their own views about the war to those at home. For Laura and Mildred, like other Canadian nurses who worked overseas, correspondence was a precious link to Canada and their families. Keeping in touch meant exchanging letters and packages, and depending on a nurse's location, delivery could be swift or slow. Letters to and from England could take as little as a week, but letters to and from remote locations such as Lemnos and Salonika could take months, with the greater distance to Canada adding to delays. Letters tended to arrive in batches and out of sequence, with packages taking even longer.[47] Such delays account for Laura and her mother's careful numbering of their letters, and the joy and enthusiasm with which mail was received, especially in isolated postings. The familiar handwriting on an envelope or a carefully chosen gift brought "home" into the war zone.

But communicating by letter across such distances and over the course of four years of tumultuous changes and experiences could, for many, cause miscommunications. Seen through Russian genre theorist Mikhail Bakhtin's notion of dialogism,[48] letters become a series of responses to previous communications, changing roles, and previous and developing cultural and educational perspectives.[49] Each writer imposes a range of selves both on herself and on her reader: such roles may correspond to familial roles, professional roles, gender roles, and other roles. Such selves can range from the "concrete to the ideal," or from the actual person to, for instance, the idealized war nurse perpetuated by public discourse through such images such as A.E. Foringer's poster of a Madonna-like nurse cradling a soldier on a stretcher in "The Greatest Mother in the World."[50] The reader, in turn, may accept or reject such imposed roles. For instance, Mrs. Holland reminds Laura, when the latter is on her first active service posting on the Greek island of Lemnos, that a nurse's gender-appropriate role in wartime is to unquestioningly accept hardships. Mrs. Holland is responding to the public discourse of soldier-heroes who may make the ultimate sacrifice in battle; a woman's role should be to accept any sacrifice or hardship as lesser. But Laura prosaically rejects such assumptions, noting that "we are all willing to put up with hardships that can't be avoided – but when it can be remedied why suffer in silence?"[51] Such assumptions and rejections can result in miscommunication – in less intimacy between writer and reader. Fortunately, Laura and Mrs. Holland, as mother and daughter, and Mildred and Cairine Wilson, as friends since schooldays, were sufficiently close that disagreements rarely occurred. Then, too, Laura's and Mildred's vivid, usually direct descriptions of their wartime lives were sufficient to counteract much of the public propaganda about their work and the soldiers they nursed.

A commonly accepted assumption about First World War letters is that the writers passively accepted the censorship regulations that governed letters home and that censorship severely affected the content.[52] My previous studies, however, have demonstrated that many war writers, including Mildred, Laura, and their colleague Helen Fowlds, actively subverted censorship regulations to maintain stronger connections with those at home, especially when patients and medical staff suffered from shortages, "refus[ing] to remain silent" even when ordered to do so.[53] Canadian nurses' letters were usually doubly censored, as were those of most war participants on active service. The first censor was an officer within the unit, who was usually known to the writers; the second was an impersonal, unknown censor at the base in England. Censorship regulations originally were put in place to prevent leaks of military information to the enemy. In 1915 cameras were banned, as were soldiers' personal diaries.[54] Gradually, regulations expanded to the point that criticizing those in authority could be construed as treason. But Laura sent a number of uncensored letters to England and Canada with returning personnel, and so felt freer to "talk" to her mother; she also found two officers at CSH No. 1 who were willing to sign her letters unread, replicating an honour system prevalent in the British army.[55] She also buried many critiques and comments deep within her lengthy letters. If at times she felt constrained, the feeling usually wore off relatively soon after reaching a new posting. Though careful to avoid most military details, she could not resist describing, for instance, meeting the first soldiers evacuated from Gallipoli or the trenches she visited while at Salonika.

But the privations nurses and their patients suffered on Lemnos with CSH No. 1 were "dangerous territory" to write home about. An international scandal threatened when reports of shortages and careless British administration reached home via letters written by medical staff, including the nurses.[56] As a result, the nurses were threatened with severe censorship in November 1915. Laura wrote repeatedly to warn her mother not to pass her letters around outside the family, stating the regulations she was supposed to adhere to but making it equally clear that they were being ignored: "It seems we are not allowed really according to military rules & regulations to discuss even the condition of our own hospital – everything except the scenery & sometimes even that is tabooed – needless to say no-body sticks to the restrictions."[57] Mildred, more circumspect, subtly wrote around the regulations while she was a nursing sister, dropping hints and using rumours to criticize the authorities on Lemnos while seeming not to do so.[58] Yet she did mostly adhere to the restrictions when she reached new postings. Her first letter to Cairine from CCS No. 2 in Belgium, for instance, when she was still a nursing sister, states near the beginning that "it is almost useless to write letters for there is very little we can say."[59] After describing the work as "hard," the camp as "very well-laid out and splendidly run," and the mosquitoes as "large and hungry," she calls her letter "stupid," continuing that "it is hard being tied down. It gives one a feeling of having nothing to say." The act of describing her work and surroundings in terms innocuous enough to pass the censor changes the "little we can say" in letters to "nothing to say." In this same letter, though, Mildred states: "One realizes the horrors of war more than ever in this place" – a constrained sentence that paradoxically conveys the depth of emotion she feels at the casualties she deals with. Despite censorship and constraint, feelings do seep through for friends like Cairine to read. Mildred's next letters are more open, narrating casualties' stories and her own pity and horror and describing the CCS as a "hot spot" from which she and Laura may not return.

An additional problem was that Laura and Mildred's unit censor on Lemnos and at Salonika discussed the contents of the nurses' letters with other personnel; in essence, their private affairs became public knowledge within the unit. As well, Matron Charleson's friends at home apparently repeated back to her what the nurses had written to their families, who in turn had talked about their letters or circulated them in their home and social circles.[60] As a result, both Laura and Mildred felt constrained when writing about their colleagues and the causes of the tensions in the unit – though Laura was much more open than her friend, especially in her uncensored letters.

Laura's and Mildred's different attitudes towards censorship can be attributed in part to their positions within the medical hierarchy: Mildred, from a powerful family and with years of experience as a nurse and administrator, looked forward to an appointment as matron and recognized the need to remain aloof from controversy, especially about her immediate colleagues, in her writings – so long as she was not herself in power. She openly and severely criticized the British administration until told not to yet, strikingly, she never once made comments, adverse or complimentary, about any of her nursing or medical colleagues (except Laura) in any of her extant letters until she was appointed acting matron of CCS No. 2 in France. Finally in charge herself, she felt free to criticize the commanding officer, the nurses who joined her unit, and their relatives. Laura, in contrast, took many risks even in her doubly censored letters. Her sense of honour caused her to omit military doings in letters that officers signed for her unread, but she had no apparent qualms about fooling the unit censor, nor did she seem to fear censure for criticizing the matron, her colleagues, the medical staff, and the British authorities. Equally, she often praised her fellow nurses.

The impact of censorship, in fact, "was contextual and varied in its effectiveness," depending on the unit, the writer, and the censors.[61] Surprisingly, neither Laura's nor Mildred's surviving letters had any information blacked out by a censor. Self-censorship, the omission or qualification of information to avoid upsetting those at home, was a different matter. For those at home, such as Mrs. Holland, Laura's Uncle George, and Cairine Wilson, letters were reassurance that the writers were safe and alive "at the time of writing"; families and friends of nurses, like those of soldiers, endured ongoing suspense about their daughters' safety and health.[62] As a result, Mildred, for instance, deliberately chose to leave her family and friends uninformed about her 1915 illness on Lemnos until she was better.[63] Laura wrote vividly about the shortages of food and water on Lemnos, but after learning of her mother's deep anxiety, repeatedly emphasized her good appetite, described actual meals to show their improvement, and commented on how "fat" she was getting. She continued to balance honesty with caution – for instance, she does describe air raids in Salonika, but after explaining the nurses' dash for the dugout, notes that "the Zeppelin wasn't near us" and dwells more on the "wonderful sight" of the "magnificent search lights all focused on the one object" than on her own danger. Her ending, with the Zeppelin "brought down without having done any damage" emphasizes the excellence of the British defences and the resulting lack of danger for the nurses.[64] Noticeably, when she and Mildred served in the "hot spot" of CCS No. 2 near Ypres, Laura omitted all mention of the frequent air raids and shelling her CCS underwent; the danger was close and very real, so she spared her mother the anxiety of knowing about it.[65]

Yet despite these seeming omissions, accounts of the war as perceptive and substantial as Laura and Mildred's double account are exceptionally rare. They are also the only pair of female friends among the Canadian military nurses whose letters remain extant and have been reunited. For depth and coverage, only *The War Diary of Clare Gass*, edited by Susan Mann, and the letters and diaries of Helen Fowlds, available online at Trent University,[66] bear comparison in publicly available accounts by Canadian military nurses.[67] Laura's and Mildred's letters, written from Lemnos, Alexandria, Cairo, Salonika, England, Belgium, and different locations in France, provide rich insights about a greater variety of hospitals and fronts than any other Canadian nurse's narrative now extant. Clare Gass, whose diary covers her four years of war service in France and England, provides a "verbal photograph album" through her diary,[68] in contrast to Laura's lengthy descriptions and analyses and Mildred's trenchant, high-level commentary. Gass provides telling glimpses of daily life as a war nurse in France, where the work could be emotionally draining and difficult but hospitals were well supplied. Laura and

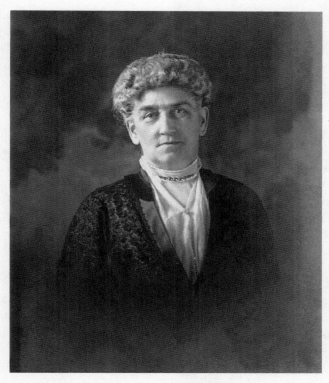

Laura Holland's mother, Laura Hadrill Holland.
Courtesy Stephen D. Cooke

Mildred convey sometimes startling contrasts to Gass's experiences in their depictions of themselves attempting to cope amid physical privations they had never previously experienced in their hitherto privileged lives – hunger, shortages of supplies for patients, and their own and their patients' depression. And Gass's diary and Mildred's letters from CCS No. 2, where Gass served under Mildred when she was acting matron, work together, providing very different perspectives: Gass contributes brief yet telling vignettes of almost unending casualties and frequent dangers, while Mildred conveys the efforts needed to maintain morale within the unit and to keep the station running smoothly, even when it is bombed out.

Helen Fowlds, a colleague and later friend of Mildred and Laura on Lemnos and at Salonika, younger in outlook and perspective than her colleagues, was, in Meryn Stuart's definition, "coming of age through these wartime experiences"; she "constructed herself as a young, modern, 'new woman' in her letters home."[69] Mildred and Laura, older, well-travelled, and mature wage earners for some years before the war, had no need to do so. Their challenge was not, like Fowlds, to see themselves as "free in a man's world"[70] for the first time, but to cope with being thrust into a patriarchal military hierarchy – a gendered hierarchy that often chafed – after years of independence. As their letters show, their close friendship sustained both women throughout challenges that sometimes threatened the perspectives, attitudes, and identities instilled by their privileged social and economic status, nursing training, and gender. As well, the contrast in their positions contributed to their different attitudes and ways of communicating their wars.

In a photograph of the staff of CCS No. 2, Mildred sits quietly and with dignity near the centre of the picture, her veil pristinely starched, her sweater elegantly draped over her uniform. Laura stands behind her and slightly to one side, her body turned towards Mildred, her face to the camera. This portrait epitomizes their professional relationship – and their personal closeness – during the war: Mildred in the foreground, Laura deliberately supportive of her friend. Mildred Forbes, related to some of the wealthiest and most influential families in Montreal, was an exceptionally able administrator and an experienced nurse and represented the best of Canadian society and of the nursing corps. These qualities would prove both a hindrance and a help in the pair's overseas postings. Mildred's letters to Cairine Wilson are written from the distinctive perspective of a capable administrator who chafes at incompetence in the military system when she does not hold power but who adheres to most regulations for the sake of discipline: she is what Cynthia Toman would call a "good soldier."[71] But Mildred is fully aware of her own abilities and enjoys using them when she has the chance to do so. As acting matron of CCS No. 2 in 1917 and 1918, she ran that important station, within the reach of the shelling at Ypres, throughout several major battles.

Laura, too, had enormous executive ability and talent, as her postwar career with the Ontario Red Cross and in social work in British Columbia demonstrates.[72] Yet as the less experienced nurse and administrator, she consciously avoided promotion during the war as her "sacrifice" for the friendship. Hers is a second unique perspective: she is both participant in and observer of the inner circles of power. Whereas Mildred's letters give the administrative perspective, Laura's provide one of the deepest, richest, and most analytic accounts of Canadian military nursing life during the First World War. From an impoverished widow in Egypt to King George V, from a tented ward on Lemnos to Matron-in-Chief Macdonald's beautiful bachelor flat, little escapes her vision. Laura's astute observations, which often question gender, cultural, and economic disparities, extend beyond the army system to the often exotic places she inhabits and the people she meets. Toman has observed that many Canadian nurses in the east "described themselves primarily in terms of whiteness, femininity, cleanliness, and British-ness in contrast to Blackness, masculinity, dirtiness, and Greek-ness," in part because of their relationship with "the British Empire's long history of dominance and privilege."[73] But Laura's intelligent observations about gender, imperialism, and the postwar future of refugees signal a developing social conscience and an openness to questioning the established order. Her war experiences clearly influenced her choice of later career and her thoughts about those deprived of power through lack of economic, cultural, or gender privileges. Where others wrote about foreign people and places as novel curiosities, Laura would write, "While one knows the goods of this world are not divided as fairly as they should be – here [in Cairo] it really worries me. [S]omehow even away out here one feels the world is topsy-turvy, & it is impossible to feel one is on a pleasure trip, even if there is no work at the moment to be done."[74]

Laura, unlike Mildred, had no compunction about breaking the "proper official silence regarding the contentious or controversial aspects of [her] war experiences,"[75] especially when she saw no sense in imposed restrictions. Where Mildred hints and is terse, Laura supplies vivid detail. Although she wrote cautiously about her nursing colleagues, her letters reveal much valuable information about the tensions between male and female officers, nurses and orderlies, and Canadian and British medical staff. Although she declares that she is "no ardent advocate for equal rights," her frequent observations about gender inequities and differences, from the Greek villagers she encounters (the women work, keeping "scrupulously clean" houses and doing the nurses' laundry, while the men "sit [in the] square and drink – drink – drink"), to men at all levels in the army, demonstrate her developing sense of gender differences and her growing sympathies for women and children living in patriarchal societies.[76] Together, Laura and Mildred's narrative of the First World War re-creates the fullness of Canadian nurses' overseas lives during it, from their professional time on the wards caring for patients to their social activities and pleasures, from their struggles with authority to their ability to wield it.

The paucity of publicly available First World War narratives by Canadian nurses partly accounts for the equally sparse references to them in international studies of Allied war nursing.[77] Even so, much sterling work has been done in Canada by war scholars in both history and literary studies. Morin-Pelletier's *Briser les ailes de l'ange*,[78] the pioneering book-length history of Canadian First World War nurses' experiences, stands alongside Toman's *Sister Soldiers*[79] as an invaluable contribution to the field of Canadian military nursing history and war studies. Previous histories are partial, from *Three Centuries of Canadian Nursing* to G.W.L. Nicholson's *Canada's Nursing Sisters*, which devotes three chapters to the First World War.[80] *On All Frontiers: Four Centuries of Canadian Nursing*,[81] contains Geneviève Allard's important chapter, "Caregiving on the Front"; it also includes intriguing short biographies of two First World War nurses, including Laura Holland. Toman has done excellent work in exploring the conflicted yet developing national identities of Canadian First World War nurses on the Mediterranean Front, and Meryn Stuart's study of Helen Fowlds's letters and diary illuminates gendered identity and construction of the "social" self.[82] Susan Mann's introduction to *The War Diary of Clare Gass* offers a fine overview of nurses' work, position in the military hierarchy, and groundbreaking overturning of traditional gender roles and authority. My own interdisciplinary study of Canadian nurses' relations with patients on Lemnos also contributes an in-depth analysis of censorship in nurses' letters and their rebellion against authorities' attempts to silence their stories of patients' needs, combining historical research with a literary scholar's reading of nurses' narratives.[83]

Laura and Mildred's double narrative of war illuminates the diverse perspectives and meanings held by Canadian nurses, and the diverse communication strategies they employed, even as they experienced the same events. Reading Laura's and Mildred's rich accounts of their wars in the context of other Canadian military nurses' writings highlights the importance of Helen M. Buss's observations about the diversity of women's writings and viewpoints. Buss points out that each new Canadian women's autobiographical narrative that we encounter "revises ... historical and cultural maps of this place."[84] When "this place" is the First World War, and Canada's memories of that war remain predominantly male, every woman's account of it adds to our knowledge and understanding of the meaning of war for Canadian women and the roles they perceived themselves playing within it.

FRIENDSHIP AND WAR

Carolyn Heilbrun, writing of the renowned friendship between British writers Vera Brittain and Winifred Holtby, tells us that "friendship between women is seldom recounted" and that when it is, it is limited to "those family crises" of "marriage, birth, death, isolation. From the love of women for one another as they work and live side by side ... recorders of civilization have averted their eyes."[85] This "continued marginality" occurred because women's eighteenth- and nineteenth-century friendships were constructed as "second best to heterosexual marriage," which offered "social and economic security."[86] Lilian Faderman observes that "early twentieth-century women ... had grown up in a society where love between young females was considered the norm," a preparatory state for heterosexual marriage.[87] By the late nineteenth and early twentieth centuries, too, female friendships, seen as "more influenced by sincere emotion than by reason, and motivated more by feeling and sympathy than by practical issues," were being used to reinforce perceptions that women's place was in the home, as wives and mothers.[88] But the "second generation"[89] of Canadian trained nurses chose economic independence outside the home; their profession, though calling for sympathy, emphasized reason and science over sentiment. Three years of arduous apprenticeship-style training and residence with fellow students naturally led to friendships based on proximity, shared ethics, and common goals.[90] Marriage was not an economic necessity for such women, though many eventually chose to marry and resign from their nursing positions.[91] For student and trained nurses, friendships took place outside the home, in the profession.

In contrast to women's friendships, male friendships have been celebrated since Greek and Roman times, and male comradeship has become a trope of the First World War. As Canadian historian Jonathan Vance explains, "friends were linked by common interests and tastes" whereas "comrades ... were joined in a common fate. The strength of their relationship lay in a shared response to the conditions they experienced at the front."[92] Male comradeship, for Canada, was one of the saving graces that took the "sting" out of veterans' memories of loss, battles, and trench conditions.[93] In contrast, Joanna Bourke's study of British soldiers argues that comradeship was enforced, imposed by military rituals and regulations. As a result, male friendships became tenuous and fragile.[94]

Not surprisingly, given the contemporary privileging of male battle experience over female war service, Janet Lee's study of friendship and comradeship among the British volunteers with the First Aid Nursing Yeomanry (FANYs) shows that they called on "the feminine appropriation of military heroism ... expressed in acts of physical courage" to justify their feminine presence in the war zone.[95] Like untrained volunteer nurses, who "saw themselves as the female counterparts to soldiers,"[96] the FANYs, also volunteers, measured themselves by male standards. But trained military nurses had no need to appropriate masculine military standards. Volunteers saw war work as temporary and extraordinary, as "'doing their bit'" for the war effort, as their brothers were doing by enlisting.[97] Trained nurses such as Laura and Mildred, in contrast, would have been working in hospitals even if the war had not occurred,[98] and they tended to record only what they saw as new or "novel" in their war letters.[99] During the war, they knew that their training and experience was essential, and they saw nursing as a gendered and distinctive profession. War acted, however, as a forcing house for nurses' friendships and comradeship, and not always positively; its rapidly changing circumstances tested individuals and units alike.

The friendship of women works on many levels in the letters of Laura Holland and Mildred Forbes, but is shown to be essential, accommodated, and encouraged in the extraordinary circumstances of war; friendship provided a trusted emotional centre that imposed stability and order on suspense and chaos. Mildred and Laura's friendship was in itself unique, yet also representative of the many strong friendships that developed among the nurses: Bertha Merriman kept a photograph of her friend, Gertrude Donkin, on her dressing table for many years after the war;[100] Helen Fowlds left Salonika to emotionally support her friend Myra Goodeve when Myra had a second brother killed in action;[101] and Katharine Wilson and Sister Willett[102] became known as the "Siamese twins" for their closeness.[103] Such intimate friendships helped the women endure the "isolation and sadness that were the realities of the front."[104]

Canadian military nurses seldom stayed at the same posting for long periods of time; they went where they were needed. Although when Matron-in-Chief Macdonald knew of friendships, she usually supported them,[105] Laura and Mildred still feared separation. Mildred's rank of acting matron of the draft of nurses who sailed with her gave her rare direct access to Miss Macdonald, and she took the opportunity to tell her "that [she and Laura] were great friends & would like ... to stay together."[106] Others were not so fortunate: Helen Fowlds, writing in early 1915, wrote that "in truly Biblical fashion one friend was taken and the other left out of every group" when half the unit's nurses were transferred.[107] Despite Macdonald's support, Laura and Mildred took no chances: Laura deliberately refused any chance of promotion so that she and Mildred could have the same hours off, and Mildred turned down the prestigious matronship of a large hospital in England because she was afraid she would be separated from Laura.[108]

Friendship was to prove vital on their first foreign posting. At the end of July 1915, when they had barely unpacked at their first English hospital, Macdonald offered them the chance to join Canadian Stationary Hospital No. 1, which was about to sail for an unknown destination in the Mediterranean. They had only "half an hour" to decide. "I didn't hesitate," wrote Laura, because "our being together meant more than everything." Mildred, too, "was dying to go, but wouldn't say so," because she thought, protectively, that the less robust Laura "couldn't stand the heat."[109] Their decision made, they left in such a hurry that they had to leave their laundry behind. They were destined for the Greek island of Lemnos, sixty miles from the Gallipoli

Peninsula and six hundred miles from Alexandria, to nurse the ill and wounded soldiers from the fighting in the Dardanelles. The British medical administration, unprepared for a prolonged campaign and caught without sufficient medical facilities, requested that three Canadian hospitals join the Mediterranean Expeditionary Force: CSH No. 5 set up in Cairo, while CSHs Nos. 1 and 3 pioneered tent hospitals on Lemnos.[110]

"It seems customary for the Eng[lish] Govt. to send a Hosp. Unit to a desert island, & make *absolutely* no provision for them," wrote Mildred to Cairine shortly after the unit arrived. "Water is very scarce.... It is not fit for us to drink – & we get a *very* small allowance for washing."[111] Food was equally scarce and unappetizing: as Laura wryly observed, "To-day @ dinner while eating, 8 [flies] fell dead on my plate from over feeding, & I have become so hardened to the sight, I don't even pick them out & throw them on the floor but just keep a grave yard in one corner."[112] The heat soared to over 100 degrees F (38 C), the winds swirled dust into the tents and wards, and most of the patients were ill with dysentery and other enteric diseases.

Friendship became essential for physical survival when dysentery swept the hospital staffs, causing the deaths of the matron and a nurse at nearby CSH No. 3.[113] Mildred contracted the disease and was confined to her tent for three long weeks, dependent on Laura – who refused to leave the camp for five weeks while her friend was ill – for nursing care. Laura wrote hopefully about Mildred's progress but could not hide her fear, juxtaposing her "up-set" and "loneliness" about Matron Jaggard's funeral and the medical personnel being invalided back to England with the story of Mildred's illness. Separation, even death, was a very real possibility. Mildred had not told her family or friends of her illness; tellingly, Laura's anxiety overcame her loyalty. Unable to express her fears to Mildred, Laura repeatedly cautioned her only confidante, her mother, to keep the secret.[114] When Laura in turn became ill, Mildred, barely recovered herself, protected her friend when their tent blew down. "The sensations I felt trying to get Lollie safely out of bed," wrote Mildred to Cairine. "We were two pitiful objects staggering out into the dark stormy night, leaving our 'home' in what seemed to be ruins."[115] Mildred's almost Gothic language reveals the strength of their bond: "home" may have been a tent, but it was a place they had created together and where they helped one another through illness and deprivation. When the nurses moved into new huts, each nurse was allotted one, but Laura and Mildred promptly created a two-hut "home," moving their beds into one hut and using the other as their living room, so creating a shared space of night-time "safety" and intimacy and a daytime space for reading, writing, chatting, and entertaining when off-duty.[116] They would follow this practice throughout the war, in Salonika, London, and Belgium.

The nurses' professional distress on behalf of their patients meant that friendship was essential for emotional stability and balance. "We can give so little to the men," wrote Mildred, "for we have so few things to work with."[117] Laura echoed her friend, writing to her mother that "it is heart-breaking ... the shortage is appalling."[118] Just as disturbing as the shortages was the discovery of the "colossal ... mis-management"[119] of military matters on the peninsula, which caused the unnecessary "sacrifice" of men.[120] Wartime medical staff built "resilience" – protection from emotional breakdown – through knowing they were constructively helping their patients.[121] In contrast, the two nurses found the work "routine,"[122] "depressing," and "un-satisfactory."[123] They could not "contain ... trauma"[124] for their patients physically or emotionally, and they could not build resilience through knowing that their training and experience were being fully used. Instead, they justified their presence through gender, by comparing the "some good" the female nurses were doing with the "awful" conditions of the hospitals run by all-male staffs.[125] Laura and Mildred's friendship became a safety valve, for they "let off steam"[126] to one another in the privacy of their tent, which helped them endure these traumas.

Though Laura and Mildred's friendship remained strong and stable, tensions among the nurses and within the hospital unit were rife, especially on Lemnos and to a lesser extent at Salonika, due to the poor facilities and scanty supplies. The army system was inherently competitive: nurses who ran wards had to requisition supplies and equipment, and those who had established good relations with quartermasters and others in charge of supplies could garner what they needed or wanted, often at others' expense.[127] The set-up of the wards on Lemnos, with each nurse on duty running her own hut as of the end of October, led to fierce rivalry for scarce supplies for patients. "The hardest fighter & worst kicker," as Laura commented, "usually [came] out on top,"[128] meaning that some nurses were able to supply their patients' needs while others went short. The aggressiveness of this infighting meant an overturning of professional and gender-appropriate behaviour: nurses' training had taught them to place the good of the hospital above the individual,[129] while loud voices contradicted ladylike behaviour. But the issue was more complicated: those who won the competition had the satisfaction of knowing that their patients were better cared for; those who lost would suffer greater emotional trauma because their patients also lost out.

Length of active war service replaced the professional status experienced nurses had gained at home: Mildred, acting matron of her draft of reinforcements in June 1915, was relegated to the newest of the new, along with Laura, because Lemnos was their first posting on active service. CSH No. 1 had been one of the first Canadian medical units organized, and it had sailed with the

First Canadian Contingent in 1914. The original nurses called themselves "the First Contingent" and took pride in their status, at times wielding it in an effort to gain prestigious positions, such as when nurses were called for to sail on a hospital ship to the peninsula.[130] This privileging caused some resentment on the part of nurses who had joined up later: Laura and Mildred, for instance, were nicknamed "The 1st Reinforcements."[131] Those who were new had to establish contacts with those who controlled supplies, struggle with army paperwork, and prove themselves on the wards and in daily life in camp.

Laura was left alone to fight for supplies for her patients and to appropriate food and drink for Mildred during the latter's long illness on Lemnos. The others had been together long enough to form friendships and cliques, but Laura knew few people in the unit and had no good friends other than Mildred. Although she did know Colonel McKee, the CO, he became seriously ill during the first week and was invalided home. This isolation would have affected her ability to obtain supplies for her patients and caused her acute anxiety because she needed food fit for her only friend. Unable to leave camp, she gave an officer £5 to obtain eatable fresh fruit, biscuits, and ginger ale; she sold some to the other nurses to provide a "treat," showing altruism even in desperate circumstances.[132]

Food was an ongoing source of tension for the nurses. Laura was "unfortunate" enough to be made mess sister during the first ten days at Lemnos and was acutely aware of her inability to perform her responsibilities satisfactorily – and of the poor impression she was making on her fellow nurses.[133] No rations had been arranged for the unit, the cooks used an open fire, few dishes or pots were available, water was chlorinated and rationed, and the little food available was unpalatable. Also, cracks appeared in her relations with Matron Charleson and the male cooks. Laura blamed the poor food directly on the matron, who "seems to antagonize everyone with whom she comes in contact," especially the men who could have arranged for shipments of food or for transport to the villages and naval ships in the harbour. She lacked "energy" and "tact" and would not allow the nurses under her (including Laura) to take over such arrangements.[134] The matron's stubbornness caused another flare-up when the nurses took matters into their own hands, pooling their funds and creating their own messing arrangements in early September, thus improving their buying power and the quality of their food while condemning their matron's efficiency by doing so.[135]

Still more friction was generated by the nurses' right of command over orderlies and non-commissioned officers. On the wards, there was "quite a bit of trouble regarding the orderlies' attitude," which led to criticism of those nurses who were the "least bit familiar with any of them."[136] Orderlies rebelled at doing the "menial work" of the ward, and "if forced to do it [did] it very badly."[137] Faced with cleaning and other jobs that women usually performed at home, the men resented nurses' orders; they refused to recognize that nurses' training and rank meant their time was better spent treating patients.

Mildred and Laura's own privileged status proved both detrimental and beneficial to them, depending on the circumstances. From the very beginning of their war service, they judged people by manners and appearance: a colonel on board ship was a "splendid organizer" but "far from being a gentleman,"[138] while the nurses at Cliveden were "indifferently nice, decidedly dull but very chatty."[139] Though both were cautious about describing the nurses at CSH No. 1, a comment Laura made about Matron Charleson is telling: "To meet socially, if one didn't know her too well, she might be alright."[140] To be socially acceptable meant having qualities that, according to Laura, the matron lacked, including appropriate clothing, emotional self-control, tact and diplomacy, altruism, and interesting conversation that did not include gossip. Noticeably, many of these qualities were those that nurse training schools had tried to instill in them, blurring the line between social acceptability and professionalism.

Paradoxically, young and attractive nurses were both lauded and condemned. The naval ships in Mudros Harbour were "a kind of wonderland" for any peninsula soldiers invited on board because of the contrast in conditions.[141] The variety and quantity of food, the china dishes, and the possibility of baths were equal attractions to the nurses – as were, for some, the attentions of young naval officers. "I don't know how we ever would have existed if it hadn't been for these naval men," commented Laura. "Of course we have several very pretty girls in our unit & that has helped more than a little."[142] The naval officers sent daily provisions for the nurses and often invited them to meals and entertainments.[143] Good looks and attractiveness were approved, then, when they benefited the collective, but considered a drawback when it came to attitude. Those "out for a good time"[144] were considered selfish for foisting their work onto others,[145] while nurses who were "young" and made regular dates with officers could be considered "flighty," their dedication to work suspect.[146]

But by 1916, Laura's judgments were based more on work ethics than on social status. Nurses who were invalided home were gauged by their dedication, their calming and beneficial influence on patients, and their skills; social judgments came second. For instance, Laura described Miss Hervey as "a good worker" with "splendid principles" after working with her; when she asked Mrs. Holland to receive Miss Hervey when the latter reached Canada, she added that Miss Hervey was "rather a peculiar, reserved woman" but with "a heart of gold" and "the disposition of a saint ... after you get to know her."[147] Laura's appreciation of character and professionalism now had priority over social capacity, in a reversal of her earlier judgments.

Few signs of *esprit de corps* are evident in any nurses' letters from Lemnos. This dearth reflects the tensions among the nurses as well as with the matron, the medical officers, and the orderlies.[148] But despite tensions among themselves, the nurses did unite on behalf of their patients. Mildred and Laura, like other nurses, made "bally nuisance[s]" of themselves with the medical staff by demanding improvements.[149] As a unit, the nurses refused to be silenced: their ethics called on them to challenge military regulations and gender barriers on behalf of their patients.[150] The nurses were also united in their desire to "make good" for Canada. At the worst of the infighting, Laura declared firmly, "Not one of us would go back if we could under present conditions." Mildred echoed her, constantly using "we" to convey the unity of the nurses in the unit and their determination to serve their patients.[151]

Above all, the Canadian nurses were united in their condemnation of the British administration's careless treatment of is own soldiers and the medical units who tended them. Mildred, angered by the nurses' treatment on Lemnos, declared in a statement echoed in other nurses' writings that "the British have only recently sent their Sisters here. I suppose by sending Australian & Canadian ones they would see how they stood it – before venturing to send their own. But we will show them ... the stuff we are made of."[152] Toman rightly argues that the nurses' "resistance" to the British "preconception" of them as "second class" resulted in a collective "emerging self-awareness of Canadian difference."[153] But as I argue elsewhere, the nurses' experience of privation, which they shared with their British patients on Lemnos and at Salonika, complicated notions of nationality: the Canadians certainly "came to a sense of distance from imperialism, which they identified as the misuse of power for troops, patients, and nurses."[154] Yet nurses also identified with their patients, the British soldiers, whom they saw as victims of the higher British authorities. As a unit, the nurses also collectively condemned any British authorities, including British matrons, who treated them as "colonials" or as second-class citizens.[155]

The "comradeship" that some other scholars claim for nurses[156] was not present on Lemnos, though the common purposes of caring for patients and of proving their own worth did unite the Canadian nurses when they spoke out against authority. Yet the daily tensions and frictions, the constant fighting for desperately needed supplies, the struggles with illness, the perceived differences in status, and the seeming lack of leadership among the nurses meant that no cohesive sense of comradeship was created. *Esprit de corps* did develop in urgent situations, such as during CSH No. 1's efforts to care for the huge influx of wounded soldiers from the 1915 Second Battle of Ypres in France.[157] But this group loyalty only developed when nurses' training and experience were valued, used, and appreciated in a crisis, which it was not on Lemnos. Comradeship did develop retrospectively[158] after the nurses had left the Mediterranean and returned to England, and it sprang from their shared experiences and endurance of harsh physical and emotional conditions. When Laura and Mildred were stationed in London in 1916 and 1917, they had tea or dinner with many of their colleagues from Lemnos and Salonika and made special trips to see others who were nursing outside London. When twelve of the "original" Mediterranean group met for tea in London, Laura commented, "You can imagine how we talked."[159] With hindsight, the frictions were forgotten, leaving the memory of challenges shared and overcome for patients and for themselves – and these bonds would last, for many, throughout their lives.[160]

Personal and professional contact eventually created bonds within the group of nurses. At the same time, letters and packages provided friendship outside the medical unit and army, with those in Canada. Letters and packages served as essential reminders of the life Laura and Mildred had left behind in Canada and that they hoped to return to, but Laura's detailed letters to her mother demonstrate her equal desire to bring her mother into her overseas life. She recorded almost every aspect of the nurses' lives, from using biscuit tins as chamber pots on windy nights, to critiquing medical inspectors, to biting descriptions of royalty. In turn, her mother and Uncle George sent news of relatives and neighbours, recorded their daily activities, and did their best to keep Laura current with changes in Canada, large and small. Their letters, throughout the war, served as preparation for her return.

Mildred, more trenchant and discreet, confessed her nostalgic longing for the "lovely peaceful" life at home.[161] But she also shared her emotions with Cairine. "One sees so many tragedies all the time that one feels positively sick," she wrote from CCS No. 2.[162] Laura was her support in the hospital; Cairine was a trusted friend in whom Mildred confided the "utter misery" of one of her patients,[163] so bringing Wilson into overseas life.

But additionally, the packages that those in Canada sent strengthened personal relationships, bestowed prestige on Laura and Mildred within the unit, and bolstered Canadian hospitals' reputations within the Allied army's medical corps. Helen Fowlds's packages from home, containing such things as underwear, stockings, and food, and her distribution of some items to her soldier brothers, "tended to fix Fowlds' identity within the family ... she remained a good, dutiful, middle-class daughter, still leaning on her parents for support

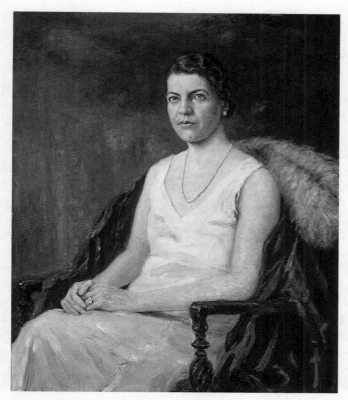

Portrait of Cairine Reay Wilson, circa 1930, by George Horne Russell. *Library and Archives Canada C-018713*

... [d]espite her status as an independent woman."[164] Most of Fowlds's packages were personal, though she did receive from her family the occasional case of goods intended for soldier-patients. Laura and Mildred's packages, in contrast, are a telling indication of their economic status and independence: Uncle George supplied whiskey, cocktails, and a lamp for their tent, while Mrs. Holland and Cairine Wilson sent luxury items such as teaspoons and glasses, olives and hors d'oeuvres, chocolates, galantine of turkey, cigarettes, soup mixes, Washington coffee, home-made candy and cakes, and underwear handmade by the Hollands' maid. These were gifts: other requests that Laura made, such as for made-to-measure boots from a Montreal store, she paid for long-distance, keeping accounts and asking her mother to take the money from her bank account, so demonstrating her status as an independent wage earner who did not expect her family to pay for her needs.

Fowlds sent "exotic ... souvenirs" to her mother, such as "Turkish brass and Belgian lace," things that would mark her travels in her "North American, middle-class home."[165] Laura felt no need to do so but spent much time in London hunting for commissions and gifts for her British-born mother and uncle: for her mother, a coat and dress and a switch (hair extension) to match her greying hair; for her uncle, menu cards and a silver biscuit box. She also sent money for special gifts such as a travelling trunk and Christmas presents, ordered flowers for her mother long-distance, and sent her a cheque for several hundred dollars.

Such a system of exchange emphasized the Holland family's stability and comfort with their social status: already a well-travelled family, they felt no need to keep souvenirs, though the luxury gifts they sent to Laura, and her return packages, emphasize their elegant manner of living and their links to their British roots. Laura justified the large cheque she sent her mother as reassurance that "in the event of anything happening to Uncle, I would love to feel that you [were provided for]."[166] But this statement comes shortly after Laura's description of another air raid. Although she rationalizes her gift through her Uncle George's potential death, it is clear that she is also concerned about her mother's future if she – Laura – is killed in a raid or dies of illness. This gift of a large sum is Laura's way of ensuring that despite the uncertainties of war, her mother will be taken care of. It also redefines the traditional mother–son, mother–daughter relationship: unlike Fowlds, the traditional, "dutiful" daughter, Laura takes the place of her brothers as her widowed mother's support.

But the packages sent through Mrs. Holland and Mrs. Wilson also endowed personal prestige on Laura and Mildred. The portable organ that Laura received acknowledged her personal love of music, but also gave pleasure to the entire unit, given that the only musical instrument they had was a badly tuned portable piano.[167] More practical gifts, such as a complete laundry kit for the nurses, baking powder (which Laura immediately turned over to the nurses' mess), a toolkit and tacks, and a baseball kit for the men in the unit,[168] would also have reflected glory on the pair and smoothed their paths. Some jealousy may have been aroused, but it would have been difficult to find fault with women who proved to be such generous benefactors through their connections at home.

Such packages for nurses and medical staff, and the many large cases of goods intended for patients, reinforced personal and professional connections beyond immediate relatives and friends. The shipments that Mrs. Holland and Mrs. Wilson organized reverberated on the nurses' personal and professional reputations within the unit, on their patients' health, and on the reputation of the Canadian hospitals. It took "endless hours [of] planning, asking and interesting people," then careful "packing," to ensure the goods arrived safely.[169] These actions created extended "families," mostly of women, within the home communities and generated personal interest in the nurses' work and their patients. Boxes sent included such thoughtful and disparate goods as towels and pyjamas for the patients, condensed milk, games and playing cards, socks, cigarettes and tobacco, powdered drink mixes, soups, medical supplies, Christmas stockings, and other goods. "When I start in thanking people for all they've done I do feel so helpless," Laura wrote, "for nothing I can say seems to give any idea of what all their thought & trouble has meant to us & the men."[170] Mildred, too, wrote about the impact of the special Christmas goods that Cairine's Red Cross chapter had made for the men in 1917, late in the war: "When I went into the tent the men were lying very dejectedly in the darkness. When the stockings appeared they bucked right up and their pleasure was a sight to behold." One "old Scotchman" even "burst into tears."[171] Such stories, told to Cairine, who would in turn relate them to her group of workers, assured the women at home that their efforts to raise large amounts of money, contribute handiwork, then collect, organize, and pack goods were boosting the nurses' professional reputations, raising the patients' morale, and helping to make the Canadian hospitals stand out among the Allied forces.[172] Both Laura and Mildred repeatedly describe the women at home as active war workers who bolstered the nurses' professional reputations and helped make "a wonderful name" for the Canadian hospitals.[173]

As the war continued, colleagues, friends, and family acknowledged Laura and Mildred as a couple; rarely did one receive an invitation without the other. When Holland's uncle visited London in 1916 and she was on night duty, he took Mildred out instead,[174] and even Matron-in-Chief Macdonald learned that Mildred was reluctant to accept invitations unless Laura was invited, too.[175] Packages sent to Laura were also designed for Mildred, as one of the family: special cocktail mixes for the two of them, and furnishings for their shared hut or tent.[176] But we cannot know, so many years later, if Laura and Mildred were lovers. Faderman claims that the concept of lesbianism was constructed as a category during the twentieth century, meaning that Laura, Mildred, and their families and friends would probably not have seen their friendship in terms of sexuality. Female friendship was unquestionably encouraged within nursing circles and in the pair's social and cultural circles. Sexual "inversion" was suspect and discouraged,[177] though "the norms of compulsory heterosexuality" within nursing made "homoerotic relations" largely "invisible."[178] In fact, anxiety about sexuality was mostly about heterosexual relationships pursued outside marriage, which might compromise Canadian nurses' reputations.[179] Certainly Laura and Mildred never constructed themselves as actively heterosexual in the way that their younger colleagues at CSH No. 1 did.[180] Whereas other nurses wrote enthusiastically about outings with officers, Laura's detailed letters focus mostly on herself and her friend. She does recount expeditions with officers, especially when the nurses were forbidden to leave camp without a male escort, but she rarely names the officers. Laura calls herself as a "really truly 'old maid,'"[181] and Mildred describes herself and her friend (at ages thirty-two and thirty-three) as "elderly."[182] Both remarks place them outside the marriage market. Younger nurses buy extravagant lingerie and uniforms, presumably as means of affirming their femininity after a hardship posting;[183] simultaneously, Laura claims that she and Mildred are the two "common sense" women in the unit – and also the "shabbiest." But she contradicts herself: both buy silk uniforms, spend hours shopping for clothes in London, and – extravagance of extravagances – purchase new evening dresses at a time when few wore them.[184] They seek to be attractive and feminine, but not to attract men. Possibly the two, loving one another, took this way of communicating to friends and relatives their lack of interest in men; equally possibly, they genuinely did consider themselves beyond marriageable age, especially given their debilitating war experiences in the Mediterranean. It is clear that other nurses used their social life and relationships with men to escape from the trauma of the wards and to re-create the social atmosphere of home. Laura and Mildred, in contrast, escaped from the war through and with one another. Not surprisingly, when the two left Salonika for England, Laura remarked, "We are enjoying to the full being off alone once more," by themselves, away from the group[185] they had been with for a full year.

If the Battle of Vimy Ridge became a male-based battle myth that supposedly created national unity within Canada,[186] then the Canadian military nurses' wartime experiences created an actual nationwide community of women, including Laura and Mildred. Working together during the war and coming in contact with nurses from across the country helped the network of nurses realize their common bonds instead of their differences. Standing with them were larger communities of women across Canada who had actively worked to uphold the nurses' work and the reputations of the Canadian hospitals. Women such as Mrs. Holland and Cairine Wilson, to whom Laura and Mildred wrote about their daily lives, their work, and their needs, represented the thousands of Canadian women who supported the nurses and hospitals, who spearheaded fundraising and drives to obtain supplies, and who took pride in their daughters and friends.

The friendship of Laura Holland and Mildred Forbes was deep and intense, made more so by the crucible of war. Together, they cared for one another through sickness and health, air raids and bombings, emotional trauma and enjoyable leaves. Yet their friendship was only one of many such throughout the Canadian nursing corps. To have a close friend in wartime meant creating stability in the midst of chaos, laughter during privation, and resilience in the face of adversity. Unlike soldiers, whose friendships could be fragile and comradeship enforced,[187] the Canadian nurses forged lasting bonds through the chaos and trauma of war.

THE LETTERS

The balance of this book presents an edited version of Laura Holland's and Mildred Forbes's letters home, divided into chapters by their geographical locations and war postings. Laura, known in her family as "Lollie," sat down on the very first day of their voyage to England to write to her mother. Her first letters, in Chapter 1, document the experience that every Canadian First World War nurse underwent: initiation into war nursing, usually by being posted to hospitals in England, as Laura and Mildred were, followed by the excitement and apprehension of a first posting on active service. Unusually, the pair were posted to the Mediterranean front instead of France. Their letters from Lemnos, in Chapter 2, movingly testify to their shock at the privations they and their patients encountered and their determination to cope. Chapter 3, about their recuperation in Cairo, highlights attitudes towards the very different cultures they encountered there, while Chapter 4 shows the two now experienced campaigners on the Salonika front, improvising iceboxes and describing air raids with humour. Chapter 5, with letters written from England after their recall in 1916, illuminates the stark contrasts between conditions in the Mediterranean and nursing in Britain. Laura and Mildred were posted to France in July 1917, arriving at CCS No. 2, near Ypres, just in time for the Third Battle of Ypres (Passchendaele). Chapter 6, the final chapter, tells of their year there, with Mildred as acting matron, then of their transfer to the more peaceful hospitals of the Forestry Corps, still in France. Laura and Mildred's war ended on May 7, 1919, when they sailed, still together, on the same ship for Canada and home. The Conclusion and Epilogue reflect on their postwar lives and accomplishments, illuminating how their wartime experiences influenced their career and life choices.

A Note on the Text

Laura Holland wrote approximately 182,000 words home to her mother in 133 extant letters between June 4, 1915, and July 12, 1917. Mildred Forbes wrote approximately 20,000 words in thirty-two extant letters to her close friend, Cairine Reay Wilson, between September 7, 1915, and January 25, 1919. (Cairine did not keep all of Mildred's letters.) To create a publishable volume, I have cut much material pertaining to personal family matters; Laura's reviews of the plays, concerts, and church services that she and Mildred attended as frequently as possible while in London; descriptions of cathedrals, cathedral towns, and other descriptive passages from Laura's and Mildred's letters while they were on leave; and much material from their time in England. Throughout the editing process, I have tried to give a balanced perspective of Laura Holland's and Mildred Forbes's experiences, development, and attitudes throughout the war years.

To create a readable narrative while maintaining the nurses' personal styles and the flavour of the times, I have indicated omissions of paragraphs and words with ellipses. In four places, I have silently moved words within sentences to make them readable. I have silently expanded abbreviations except where the meaning was clear in the original. Nurses tended to use dashes instead of commas and periods, but because readers found the original text difficult to navigate, I have silently edited punctuation throughout. I have added no unmarked words, and have retained the original sense wherever small marked deletions have been made.

I have changed all instances of "could'nt," "would'nt" and similar words to "couldn't" and "wouldn't," because readers found these spellings distracting. I have not, however, changed Laura's use of hyphens in words such as "to-morrow," feeling that these spellings give the sense of the time. Similarly, I have left words such as "un-doubtably" unchanged. I have silently corrected the spelling of words to clarify the sense, but I have not changed British, Canadian, or American versions of words. I have silently corrected some misspellings of some nurses' names. Letter and diary dates and place names in headings have been regularized. Finally, underlining in the letters has been changed to italics.

Throughout the editing process, I have endeavoured to do justice to Laura and Mildred by leaving their voices and meanings distinct and unchanged.

I

Journeying to War

Less than a month after the *Lusitania* was sunk by a German U-boat with great loss of life, Laura and Mildred sailed from Montreal to Portsmouth, England, with Mildred the acting matron of the draft of reinforcement CAMC nurses. The unexpected length of the war and the heavy casualties from bombardments and attacks meant that more hospitals and nurses were needed.

Once they arrived in London, Mildred was kept busy by Matron-in-Chief Margaret Macdonald organizing the reinforcement nurses' postings to hospitals, while Laura waited patiently or helped her friend. Thrilled at being in London, yet increasingly impatient to get to work, the pair revelled in theatres, concerts, and cathedrals, knowing that once overseas, they might have few such opportunities. Because of Mildred's position, the two were the last to be posted; despite Miss Macdonald's promise to try to place them at a hospital in France, they were first sent to an English hospital, the Duchess of Connaught's Red Cross Hospital on the Astors' estate of Cliveden, just in time to meet King George, Queen Mary, and Queen Alexandra. But after a mere two weeks there, they accepted a much greater challenge: the chance to nurse the casualties from Gallipoli and the Dardanelles.

Letter No. 1
R.M.S. Metagama
June 4th, 1915

... Dear Mother,

It is now 2.30 p.m. & can hardly believe it was this morning that I left 47 St. Mark Street. Mildred has been busy ever since she came on board, it seems to me. Had to report almost immediately to the Colonel in charge ... who although business-like was very nice; then of course she had to see the Steward about our places at the table.... Drill has been called for 3 p.m. so no time is being lost.[1] I think the Colonel fears our all being overcome with sea-sickness & so wants to have everything in good running order before any of us disappear. Of course being the first day out there is an air of confusion & up-set everywhere, & judging by the number in the dining salon, think the boat is frightfully crowded.

...

Well dear there were heaps of things I intended to say before leaving, but suppose I have too much "Holland reserve" ever to find the right moment; I'm really awfully pleased to be on the way towards helping, but hate leaving you behind, especially as I feel you've none too cheerful a time ahead of you. However let's hope it won't be for long.

Mildred sends love, & says she doesn't feel cheerful enough to say more – the responsibilities are weighing somewhat heavily I imagine, owing somewhat to un-certainty as to what is expected.

Well good-bye for the present. Take care of yourself & get a little rest, for you've been frightfully over-worked getting me off.

Lovingly yours Lollie.

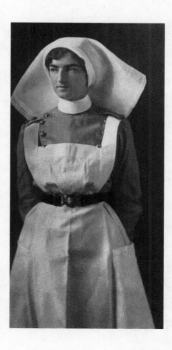

Laura in uniform, circa 1915. *UBC Archives 123.1/2*

R.M.S. Metagama
June 9th, 1915

My dear Mrs. Holland,

As Lollie is writing to you at the present moment I don't want to repeat any of her news. But I just wanted to tell you how splendidly "Mothersills"[2] is acting – Lollie will certainly have to send them a testimonial with one of her new photographs.

It was such a pity that Lollie should have got one of her headaches the first day for it certainly handicapped her. However she is drilling away and from all appearances seems fairly well.

Our life is very strenuous on board this boat, and in many ways that helps to pass the time. Lollie will have told you all about our Military manouevres[3] etc. The Colonel is a clever Military man – splendid organizer, but far from being a gentleman, & that explains a good deal.

We are all preparing for the worst to happen. It really is a wise precaution – when I arrive home I shall never feel properly clothed without a life belt adjusted on me.

Lollie & I are beginning to worry in case we are separated on the other side. Personally I would rather be torpedoed than have that happen. But everything so far has gone our way – so we can only hope that our luck will remain with us.

We manage to get off quietly for a smoke & read sometimes. At present I am the only one enjoying Mr Hadrill's whiskey, but I hope to leave some for Lollie.

Please remember me to Mr. Hadrill & with much love to yourself – and remember I will always take the best care I can of Lollie.

Affectionately yours,
Mildred

Letter No. 3
Kingsley Hotel, London
June 15th, 1915

Dear Mother,

So much seems to have happened the past two days I can't believe it was only yesterday morning we left the boat. I posted a letter to you before landing & am not quite sure where I left off. We reached Plymouth Harbour on Sunday evening but were not allowed to land. Got up Monday at 5 a.m.,

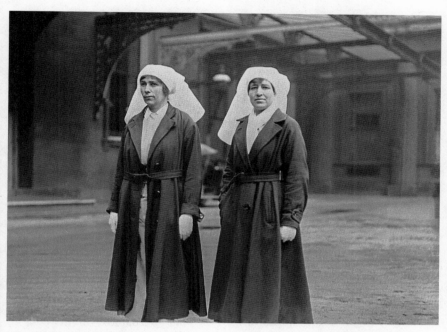

Nursing Sister N.J. Onright, RRC, and Nursing Sister Mildred Forbes, RRC.
Canada, Dept. of National Defence/Library and Archives Canada

breakfasted at 6, & then as usual had to wait around expecting to land any moment. Finally at about 7.45 a.m. a tender came along & took us ... on board ashore. The sail up the harbor or sound ... is simply beyond description. The shore is most picturesque, & as you keep quite close to land one is able to really see it....

No one met us, & finally after waiting around for an hour, a transportation Officer came along & thought we ought to go to London, so we walked to the station, a distance of about 1/2 a mile, where we saw another Officer who made arrangements for us to go on the 10.30 train. We all travelled 1st class, having lunch on the train, & arrived in London at 3.10 p.m. It was a lovely trip through the most beautiful country, and of course everything is looking its very best this season of the year. I just longed to get out & walk along some of the beautiful roads we passed. If one could manage it, certainly coming by way of Plymouth is an ideal entrance into England.

While waiting for lunch, Mildred & I happened to pass a few remarks to an Englishman & his wife (Londoners), & afterwards had a most interesting talk with them. He is a manufacturer of ammunition & it was most interesting to hear the English point of view. As far as news goes they evidently get a good deal less than we do, & while a great deal of ours may not be true, even so I think we get a better idea of the situation of affairs than the general public does here. Everybody seems to be on the lookout for a *gas* raid here, & the stores are full of respirators of all kinds, & apparently a great many people are investing in them by way of preparation.

Well to go back to our arrival, through some hitch no one met us in London, so Mildred phoned the Canadian Headquarters, the 50 of us in the meantime *waiting* on the platform per usual. Finally she got hold of someone, who was most apologetic & told us all to go to either the Kingsley or Thackeray Hotel. Mildred & I are at the former. We arrived here feeling very dirty & rather tired, having been on the way since practically 6 a.m. However we cleaned up a bit, had dinner, & the two of us rushed off to the Alhambra, feeling there was more chance of a seat there than at any of the regular theaters. Also I was rather keen to see Gaby Deslys. The greater part of the programme was taken up with the Revue – in one sense a disappointment. The gowns, chorus & staging were exquisite but there was nothing to it otherwise. Gaby herself wore gorgeous gowns & danced beautifully when she danced at all, but she spent too much time talking to satisfy me. However we enjoyed it....[4]

This morning right after breakfast we took a taxi down to Victoria Street where we had to report. As Mildred had a bunch of papers to carry, we couldn't go on a bus. Miss Macdonald,[5] the C.A.M.C. in charge, is a Major, & beyond Mildred is too grand to speak to any of us. The whole morning was wasted waiting around to sign more papers.... Then Mildred & I had to look up some lost luggage, & while everyone at the station was most polite & attended to our wants very quickly, it all took time.

The afternoon we spent in the shops. We had one or two "extras" to get such as a panama hat.... Of course [we] wasted no end of time gazing in the shop windows. We did Bond Street, Regent Street, Oxford Street, & really covered a lot of ground. I invested in a birthday present for you, but am not quite sure what to do with it.... Now shall I send it by post & risk duty, or shall I keep it on the chance of someone going across? Shall *wait* until I hear from you before doing anything.

There were so many things I wanted to buy & send home, but just had to resist all temptation for my money seems to be flying. However once we get settled it will be easier. It was fairly late when we had finished, & having made up our mind to stay in for the evening, as Mildred had a lot of papers to see to, we walked along & had a look at Buckingham Palace. Of course all that district is entirely changed since we were here and the Avenue leading up to Queen Victoria's Memorial is magnificent.[6] From there we walked through St. James Park to Piccadilly near Half Moon Street & from there took a bus home.

...

In some ways, largely because we know so few people, we seem less conscious of the war here than at home. On the other hand I feel sure any old timer would see a tremendous difference. Soldiers of course are everywhere. In St. James Park temporary wooden buildings are erected for offices of various kinds in connection with relief work, recruiting etc. Many of the grand houses are apparently being used for hospitals & convalescent homes. But ... the shopping district remains the same, & the residential districts have the usual lovely window boxes – they seem to me even brighter & gayer than before. It is not really so dark at night as I anticipated. There are no glaring advertisements, & no doubt fewer street lights.... All have a covering of some kind on top, & the light shines only downwards. Then the theatres all seem to be using rather soft colored lights outside, instead of the usual blaze.

I don't seem to have told you half of what I wanted to but you'll have to read between the lines for it's time for me to go. Soon no doubt we'll be at work & these few days will be a dream, but a mighty nice one.

My love to Uncle George. Tell him I was surprised to find how at home I felt around Oxford Street.

I'm longing to get a letter but of course it's too soon yet. I do hope you are feeling more rested. I feel we almost worked you to death before leaving. I sometimes wonder [how] I manage to get along when I leave home, for you always do so much for me.

Well au revoir for the present. Will write again soon. Heaps of love always

from Lollie ...

Letter No. 4.
London
June 20th, 1915

Dear Mother,

Of course per usual the right moment for letter-writing never seems to arrive.... In some ways a good deal of time gets wasted meeting Mildred (she has to report each morning) & nearly every day there is some business to be attended to in connection with our bunch of nurses, and I always go with her. However we are benefiting so much through her being Matron that even if we only get the afternoon or evening to do exactly as [we] please ... feel we

have no right to grumble. It seems funny when one hears of the amount
of work to be done in France that they have so much difficulty finding
places for us – but evidently nothing is done in a hurry; on the other hand,
we might be sent off on six hours' notice. However Miss Macdonald, the Matron-
in-Chief, told Mildred that she, being Matron, would be the last of the lot
to leave London. So far only 21 have been sent off, 10 to Shorncliffe, & 11
to Clivedon.[7] Mildred has of course told Miss Macdonald we are great
friends & would like ... to stay together, and there appears to be every
chance of it.

...

None of the girls in England seem to be working very hard, but the McGill
girls[8] are of course anxious to get their own Hospital, & hope to do so by
July 1st. Miss Jack[9] & Doss Cotton[10] are also at Clivedon – likewise Martha
Allan,[11] evidently very much to the fore, but so far not allowed to do much
nursing; is kept busy I believe sorting linen, making dressings etc.

...

Everyone here seems to think the War will last indefinitely. Am longing
for a letter, but imagine from all accounts the mail is frightfully mis-managed.

...

I wonder if Uncle knows Alfred Temple[12] is at the front. Evidently some
army medical corps. He is running an ambulance motor, and is right in the
thick of things....

Well dear once again good-bye. I suppose by the time this reaches you
Temple will be home. My love to him & Uncle George.

Heaps of love always to your own self

From Yours lovingly
Lollie.

[P.S.] ...

Letter No. 5
Kingsley Hotel, London
June 25th, 1915.

Dear Mother,

I can't believe this is Friday, & I haven't sent you a line since Sunday. In
some ways have had to waste a good deal of time this week one way & another, but feel so lucky at being kept in London so long, that I've no right to
grumble.... As Miss Macdonald ... seems to like Mildred, there is every
chance of our being kept together.

...

I don't know whether I've mentioned how comfortable we are here. Curiously enough the people in the Office have been rather snippy & certainly have not treated us as though we were ordinary guests, so Mildred lost her temper the other day, & feeling hot, complained to Miss Macdonald, who was furious, for she says it is a splendid thing for a hotel of this type to get the nurses as ... there is little tourist trade these days. So this morning the Manageress ... asked to see Mildred, & she couldn't have been nicer, though apparently she felt Mildred might have complained herself. However as Mildred said, it was not military etiquette & she could only complain through her superior. The maids have all been alright, it is just the office. It's the old story of nurses in this country being treated like servants! But it does make you mad.

...

Always love to you from Lollie.

[P.S.] ...

Letter No. 8
London
July 7th, 1915

Dear Mother,

...

... On Monday we stopped in front of the Exchange Building & heard some of the recruiting speeches. You know they are having a big campaign here this week, & really the whole thing makes one feel almost humiliated. It seems the recruits are not coming in as anticipated, so now all the speakers are taking a threatening attitude, & telling the crowds that unless they come in now voluntarily, just as soon as Lloyd George gets the output of munitions to exceed the men, then there is to be Conscription[13] when they will be taken by the collar & forced to join, & be compelled to wear a different uniform stamping them as Conscript men, etc, etc. This attitude seems necessary with the lower classes, but it makes one feel sick to hear it. I hate conscription in theory, but certainly over here one sees the necessity for it in time of war, for the class of people who ought to go are not doing so. They say 75% of the men who have joined are married men between the ages of 28 & 38, averaging three children in each family....

Don't read all this to the family – but thank goodness I don't have to earn my living over here! I noticed the class distinction when here before, but much more so this time. I'm inclined to think perhaps our uniform has something to do with it, for it stamps us as nurses, & of course a nurse has no standing at all.... It's this attitude that makes me want to go to France. ...

Love to the family – a whole heap always for yourself from Lollie.

Letter No. 11
July 21st, 1915.
Duchess of Connaught
Canadian Red Cross Hospital
Taplow, Bucks

Dear Mother,

So much seems to have happened since I wrote you last Friday afternoon that I don't quite know where to begin.

As you see we are at Clivedon, rather to our surprise as the Matron-in-Chief had told us we would go to France, but found it at the last impossible to arrange. Of course I have hardly spoken to her Highness, but she has been awfully decent to Mildred, & even now feel when the opportunity offers, we will be sent off. In the meantime, especially at this season of the year, we couldn't come to a nicer spot than Clivedon. However mustn't skip ahead so quickly, but go back to Saturday.

In the morning reported with Mildred, or rather per usual waited outside while she did so. Then hearing we were to go on Monday went with Mildred to see about one or two things.... The afternoon was wet & cold, so only went to see the big Woman's Procession. Expect you read all about it in the paper. I believe it was considered a splendid turn-out, certainly there were plenty of them, but they were far from attractive. In spite of the wind & the rain, many had on white dresses [and] shoes ... so you can imagine the be-draggled effect! and on the whole they appeared decidedly beneath what is known in England as the middle-class.

... In the afternoon we went to the London Opera House to hear "Madam Butterfly." It was most beautifully put on. The scenes were perfect ... Queen Alexandra was there – in the distance looks wonderfully young & attractive, her manner seemed so bright & interested; but I saw her at close quarters to-day & the shock was great.

She visited the Hospital to-day, & I was very close for several minutes – somehow she struck me as being pathetic. Her complexion is wonderful, but even through a heavy veil one can see her eyes are those of an old woman, &

her mouth the same. Her voice sounds very weak & quavery, she has the actions & smile that so many deaf people have, she is quite lame, & walks like an old woman – all this with fair hair & pink & white complexion seems pathetic. It seems a pity she didn't at some time adopt the old-lady, with gray hair etc. She would have gained rather than lost. However I must say her manner was most gracious, & if it hadn't been for Mrs. Astor, who kept hurrying her along, she would have shaken hands with every patient in the place. She motored up from London with the Princess Victoria (who looks half witted) & the Princess Royal, who appears very delicate, thin & old....

...

[On] Monday we took the 2.15 train down & per usual were not met. After some time a big bus came for us & we reached the Lodge or Nurses Home, where we sat for an hour or so before the Matron came, when we had tea, & sat around aimlessly until dinner time after which the Matron showed us our rooms & had our luggage taken there.

Mildred & I are in a large room on the ground floor with eight beds in it & six small screens. There are five large French windows so we get plenty of air, & in the evening are allowed a grate fire, so really are most comfortable, though they say in wet weather it is frightfully damp. In the meantime it's mighty nice – the only problem is getting washed. It's somewhat of a fight to get near any water in the a.m. or p.m. either for that matter.

It is hopeless trying to write, for the others in the room, indifferently nice, decidedly dull but very chatty, keep on making remarks, & reading out scraps from their home paper. There is a small sitting room, but it is worse than here – for the Officers use it as well, that is those who are interested in any of the girls.

Well Monday morning we were all excitement as to where we would go. I drew the operating-room much to my regret, for it is decidedly more inter-esting to be with the men in the wards – on the other hand the work is much lighter. We probably will have some hard days, but on others get a chance to do more or less as we like.

Altogether it was a record day. The Hospital received a batch of new patients, 200 in number. The train reached Taplow at 12.20, a distance of 2 ½ miles from the Hospital, & every man was *bathed*, clothes changed, & in bed by 3 p.m. with the Wards as neat as a new pin. The rush was on account of a visit of the King & Queen, who arrived to the minute. I was sent to a Ward in the afternoon to help out, as nothing was doing in the operating room.

The King ... is small, but wonderfully healthy looking. He was awfully nice to the men – stopped & spoke to almost everyone in the ward I was in, the Queen following & doing the same. Of course we had a splendid chance to see them.

We go on duty at 8 a.m. & get off at 8 p.m. & [are] supposed to have 3 hours off but of course on a day like this couldn't.

Certainly the work here [is] not anything like as hard as private-nursing, & even in France ... while they have terrible rushes at times, in-between whiles the work quiets down. Well I'm rather tired, & we have a big day ahead of us to-morrow in the operating room, so had better get to bed. I just wish I could get hold of you & tell you about things but ————

Mildred has a dreadful cold & is feeling generally rotten. She is in one of the Medical Wards.

... Being with the men makes me realize the awfulness of the *War*. It is pitiful to see how *every one* of them dread the possibility of ... having to go back.

Good night & heaps of love to all especially yourself from
  Lollie.

Meals are A.I.

Letter No. 12
Clivedon
July 25th, 1915

Dear Mother,

...

  I think I mentioned the Lodge ... has been turned into a Home for the nurses, & part of it for the use of the Doctors, all of whom have tents in front, with the exception of our O.C., an Ottawa man.[14] ... [F]rom all accounts, [he] is a good organizer, but seems to have nothing else to his credit. I have not spoken to him, but no one seems to like him from the Officers down, & certainly to look at he is most un-attractive. Very ordinary, makes rounds *chewing gum*, & altogether a mighty poor representative of any country. He treats all the nurses abominably, I believe, the Matron included,[15] & as she is a woman with but little dignity & not specially capable, can't hold her own against him at all – consequently the nurses suffer more or less for it. It does seem too bad that a Hospital which seems perfect in almost every other way should have two such heads – however such is life.

  Our mess is run by the nurses themselves, & certainly the food is awfully good....

The Lodge is really a very pretty house, & has been I imagine well furnished, for some of the pictures are very good, ... bits of beautiful china [are] around, & in the dining room, the walls are entirely covered with beautiful tapestry & the fireplace & doors are exquisitely carved. Upstairs there are numerous bed-rooms, some holding two, others three, four & five beds.

I am in the "ball-room," surrounded by large mirrors & French windows. Of course with eight beds & cheap little bureaus, the room looks rather a muddle, but ... the ... chintz curtains & ... screens, covered with bright pink roses, make the room cheerful. It is frightfully damp, & even this time of year cold, but we are allowed a fire each afternoon & so spend most of our time in here, leaving the drawing-room for the girls who are special favorites with the officers. I know the latter too little to make any comments....

We have about [a] 4 to 5 minute walk to the Hospital, which in wet weather is beastly, & since arriving haven't had a day but rain-coats & umbrellas were necessary. Not that the rain is continuous, but alternate hours of sun-shine & heavy rain, which keeps the grounds & everything damp. My! but I hate the thought of winter!!!! Flannels for me I know – I haven't made up my mind as regards cashmere stockings.

I think I told you the first or main part of the Hospital is the old "squash" or in-door tennis house. The main part has been divided into four wards & one of the side rooms has been made into an operating-room, behind both of which has been added lean-to or kitchen. The rest of the hospital is a series of narrow long wooden huts, with splendid bathrooms to each one. Each hut is divided into two wards, containing 50 beds each. So far there is only accommodation for 500 but when finished we will have room for 1200 patients.

...

So far we have had very few Canadians, not more than 15 or 20 out of the 500, which we rather regret, for the men are unanimous in saying they are treated far better in every way in all the Canadian Hospitals than the British, with ... regards food, & by the Doctors.... This is no doubt largely due perhaps to the fact that ... the English Doctors are stricter on the subject of Military discipline, but ... thought that *that* attitude was dropped somewhat when invalided.

I am longing to go [on] some of the walks around here, & on the river which runs right through the estate ... but will have to wait until we are out of quarantine.[16]

...

In spite of being here we feel much further from the war than when at home. Hardly even get the daily news.... Love to Uncle & a whole heap for your own self

      from Lollie.

Letter No. 13
London
July 30th, 1915

Dear Mother,

Time is so limited & I am so excited & tired after rushing around all day, I don't quite know where to begin.

...

Thursday & Friday were both very busy days in the operating room, & on the afternoon of the latter got word from the Matron that if Miss Forbes & I wanted to go to the Dardanelles to send word immediately. We were given half an hour to decide. I didn't hesitate, for I felt the next place offered we might not like & would feel bound to accept, whether we would be together or not, & the fact of our being together meant more than everything. Mildred was dying to go, but wouldn't say so, for she felt I couldn't stand the heat. However in the end we both decided that if we refused we would in all probability regret it, so sent word by the Colonel & last night at 8 p.m. got word to come to London this morning, so got busy & packed, quite a job as we had settled down in Clivedon we thought for weeks. However here we are minus only our laundry, but live in hopes it may follow us to-morrow.

Miss Macdonald on reporting this morning would not tell us where we were bound for, & is not quite sure when we leave, but said we must be all ready by noon to-morrow. Had orders to get lustre coats at Shoolbreds, (for which they soaked us £5) & they are the worst looking things you ever saw. However we hadn't time to fuss, & had to get the regulation thing. Also have been ordered to get white shoes & stockings, so far have failed to get anything near my size, Mildred also; the shops seem sold out. We were ordered numerous other small things, & strongly advised ... to get riding skirts, so as nothing in that line can be had ready-made in khaki, we left our measurements & are having them follow us a week later.... For this we had to pay 2 £ ... but as I say we just had to take what they offered. They are made so as to be used as walking skirts as well, & as our cloth uniforms will be un-wearable in the East, they are sure to be a comfort.

From there I went & had a shampoo – & as usual lately had hard luck. They took two hours of my precious time doing it & when I went to bed at night found it so greasy from some stuff they had used, had to go back & have it done again this morning. Such a waste of time!! Last night, feeling ... we could do nothing further regarding equipment until next day, rushed off to see H.B. Irving & Lady Tree in "The Angel in the House" but it was a very poor show, & we would have been wiser to stay at home & [start] to pack.

This morning as I said, I had to get my hair done again, Mildred going to the Bank. We are to go to Shorncliffe this afternoon, spend the night there & leave at 6.45 a.m. Sunday for Southampton, where we go off in some boat to parts un-known. Rumour says we go to the Island of Lemnos but ———
...

Miss Upton & Galt[17] I believe are joining the Hospital we are to be attached to. It is ... No. 1 *Stationary* Hospital....[18]

This letter is an awful scrawl, & my mind more or less in a whirl, it has all been such a rush. I said in my cable we had two days here, but it hasn't been more than 1 ½ & as you know, the distances are great.

Good-bye for the present. Heaps of love dear – & don't worry if my letters for a while are frightfully irregular.

> As always, Yours lovingly
> Lollie.

> Letter No. 14
> Folkestone
> July 31st, 1915.
> 11.15 p.m.

Dear Mother,

So far so good – & in many ways feel we have been most fortunate.

Travelled down from London with about 75 nurses, only four however belonging to our unit, No. 1 Stationary Hospital. On arriving we were sent to the ... [Métropole] Hotel where our unit are staying. A Miss Charleson is our Matron, & to my delight & surprise find Colonel McKee is our Commanding Officer.[19] It is not that I like him so much, but knowing him makes such a difference, & he was awfully nice. Also spoke to Dr. Bauld & find he is one of our unit also. Certainly life is full of surprises.

... Just spoke to Galt for a minute & believe Upton is somewhere around. I wonder if sending three of the Canadian Hospital Units to the Mediterranean means that some of our troops are going there. I imagine so.[20]

I feel we are very poorly equipped for a hot climate, where we had planned for a cold winter in France, also our laundry is in Clivedon, & our trunk is full of dirty clothes. But such things can't be helped. I seem to have spent a lot of money too.

Mildred & I have a very grand room – this is I imagine a first class Hotel, one of the best here – & we haven't even a tooth brush, & will have to sleep in our skirts!!! Major Patch didn't allow us hand bags & we stupidly let our hold-alls go with the other luggage.... Am going to hunt up someone & borrow.

Well we feel a bit tired having been on the go since 8 a.m. & it is always rather worrying, trying to get things done in a hurry. But once on the boat will have ten days complete rest. Have invested in two boxes of Mothersills, for I am told we are apt to have a good deal of rough weather.

I wish I could be there when you open my cable. Am sure it will be a surprise.

Give Uncle my love & tell him his letter was a great treat & will be answered once I am on the boat.

Am rather afraid this may not reach you in time to wish you many happy returns of August 10th but it will let you know I am thinking of you that & every day, & may we spend your next birthday together....

Once again good bye & just heaps of love to you from
    Lollie.

P.S. We have breakfast in the morning at 5.45 so are to have an early start. Once again good bye. Am afraid it will be a long time before I have another letter from you....

Letter No. 16
R.M.S.P. Asturias
August 8th, 1915

Dear Mother,

...

    I am just beginning to realize what a long distance we are from home – imagine not getting an answer to this for nearly three months!! We have all decided already that Xmas presents from home will be out of the question, though once we definitely get settled somewhere, probably our mail won't be so un-satisfactory as we imagine.

...

August 11th
Alexandria Harbour[21]

The excitement all day has been intense, & it's difficult just to know where to begin. I awoke this morning to find we had anchored about 5 o'clock in Alexandria Harbour, but hearing we would probably remain here for several hours before landing, did not rush about getting up. Had breakfast at 8 a.m. After lunch the Colonel, having received no orders ... got tired of waiting & with the O.C. of the boat ... went to shore....

On seeing Alexandria from the ship, we all were most enthusiastic & delighted we were coming here, instead of landing at Malta. The Harbour is most picturesque, & the buildings in the distance like a piece of stage scenery, so perfect & typical of pictures one has seen of the East, with occasional palm trees dotted here & there. There are boats without number in the Harbour, dozens of brigs & schooners belonging to the enemy & interned for the time being, several war-ships, hospital ships, passenger boats etc., & of course a constant stream of small yachts & small sailing vessels with those picturesque large curved sails. Fortunately for us, we again have a cool breeze blowing, & while it is *hot* it is not un-bearable.

Well to proceed with the news. The Colonel having departed, who should arrive on the scene but some naval man with the orders, & you can't imagine the disappointment & excitement caused by the announcement that No. I & No III ... were to proceed to Lemnos, a small island 40 miles from the Dardanelles. You can't imagine the shock, for while it had been whispered as a possibility when in London, the officers on this boat said it was an impossibility, for no women could be sent there. They had told us fearful tales about the place, a few of which have since been contradicted, so won't repeat as they may be wrong.

Well, all kinds of rumours have been going the rounds, but finally Colonel McKee has returned & confirmed the report, so evidently we are to go; but he also added that it is considered cooler than here, so my spirits immediately rose.

No. 5 Stationary Hospital (... Queen's from Kingston) are to go to Cairo, & while at first we were terribly envious of them, after all we will see more from a professional point of view & anyway we've no choice so why grumble.

I'm not going to tell you all the rumours about the place, for they vary too much.... But all agree no European women have been there, so we ought to create somewhat of a sensation.

It is now 5 p.m. & there is, I am afraid, no chance of our landing to-day, but we hope to do so in the morning, & Colonel McKee says we will probably remain here until Saturday. I believe we are to be transferred to another boat, much to everyone's regret.

We are all beginning to feel quite exhausted after our day of un-rest, though we have done little except lean over the rail looking for news & seeing what there was to be seen. In fact this is the first time I have sat down to-day.

Each day we feel more & more the ways of Military life are strange. You are rushed off without proper equipment & land somewhere to find you are not expected, & waste time waiting for orders, when you long to be out getting necessaries. There was talk of sending us on immediately but Colonel McKee has insisted on some time for he says the men must have different clothing.... [A]t present they have nothing but flannel shirts & heavy uniforms – in fact what they have been wearing all winter in France.[22]

I simply can't realize I am away off here in the East – even this glimpse is of the greatest interest – & while the day may come when we will regret the day we had to come to a hot climate, at present it seems well worthwhile, & judging by reports we are badly needed. Imagine Alexandria being practically the nearest hospital, over two days journey! I believe there are two hospitals at Lemnos for those who are only slightly wounded, who will probably return shortly to the front, but there are no nurses.

...

Heaps of love dear, & don't worry about me – so far haven't minded the heat much, so live in hopes it won't be too bad. Once September arrives anyway it starts to get cooler.

...

    Yours lovingly
      Lollie.

[P.S.] ...

R.M.S. Delta
August 14th, 1915

Dear Mother,

In my last letter I told you about having arrived in Alexandria on the 11th – on the 12th we had permission to go to town about 10 a.m. but by the time we got sufficient boats to take us to shore ..., it was fairly late, then we had to hunt up cabs ..., as we were a long way from the shopping district. Our Matron came in our rig, & consequently she was attached to us all day, which delayed matters more than I can say – but she's so far been decent to us, so here's hoping it may continue....

Our driver tore through the streets in the most reckless manner; I thought every minute we should be thrown out. He couldn't speak a word of English, so it was useless to remonstrate. We went through I imagine what would be considered the slums of even Alexandria. But it really is wonderful, & brings to mind continually Bible stories. One no longer is surprised at Christ having been born in a stable, for apparently that is the only place the poor live in. The buildings have the appearance of being dwelling houses & you see inside a regular stable, & the members of the family live on the streets & only go inside to sleep. Through this part you see no Europeans at all.

It is impossible in one letter to give an idea of all we saw even in that one short day. The squalor, dirt, smell, poverty, tumble down ... houses, dust & heat, & yet in spite of it all the wonderful picturesqueness of the whole. The brown men in their many colored clothes, the wonderful way they carry themselves, throw themselves down to rest in all kinds of corners & places in the most graceful positions, & yet they appear most insolent. And then there are the black men, many in rags – the veiled women. As I say it is too much to describe.

...

We passed one little kid in the door-way asleep, just a picture, & it gave you the creeps to see one of the men passing, slink up & put his hand inside the youngster's shirt & steal some treasure he had in a bag. Several saw him do it, but beyond smiling, took no notice. It is all such a mixture of picturesqueness, roguery, & filth, it positively makes one feel ill.

... [F]inally we arrived in the shopping district, where one came in contact with roguery but in slightly more respectable clothing. The shops are the queerest mixture of all that is modern & the reverse. One gets such surprises. We had to waste time while Miss Charleson bought various things, as the Colonel had said no nurse was to appear on the street alone, & amongst other things she needed boots, & do you know we could get much better looking ones here than in England. Also we had the most delicious ice-cream & iced coffee I've ever tasted even in our own country – & the following day, I got my hair shampooed in a French shop in the most luxurious (if rather expensive) fashion. They use a wonderful moveable basin with running water & waste pipe, which you use as a pillow (more or less), & they work from behind.

... [W]e shopped like mad until 12.30 noon (when they close until 3 p.m.), getting numerous necessary odds & ends, as we heard at Lemnos we couldn't

even buy a hairpin. Then had sand-wiches & the most delicious cakes in a
French pastry shop, took a cab & drove out to some Gardens.... Everything
has rather a dried-up look ... but the acacia trees are beautiful, so green,
feathery & healthy looking, some covered with the most exquisite blue
blossoms. Being some big festival day, everyone was out in holiday attire,
& the crowds were immense, but it is surprising ... how few Europeans are
around; we saw *none* outside the shopping district, & then they were either
men in khaki, or a French speaking people, & very few of the natives knew
a word of English....

When we got back from our drive I was about all in, for the heat was
beyond description, but we got one or two things, (it's like dragging teeth to
really decide on a price for anything & get out of a shop), had a cup of tea
& drove down to the wharf (there are miles of it) ... [W]ere told our boat
had finally docked; then we had some difficulty in finding where, but finally
arrived ... laden with parcels to discover ... our trunks & hold-alls had been
transferred to another boat in spite of only being half packed.... However
such is active service.... The following morning ... we were given permission
to go to town on condition we were back at sharp 12 – so I rushed off to a
hair dresser with Mildred, & had the shampoo I spoke of. We had an extra
early lunch expecting to go off to another ship immediately, but owing to
several delays, we stood on the deck, our parcels beside us, until the dinner
gong went!!!! But finally we went at 7.30 p.m. to another Hospital Ship called
the Delta, while our officers & luggage went on another boat, Colonel McKee
coming, though, to look after us, T.G.

The orders are to proceed to Mudros Bay, Lemnos Island, but whether we
land there or not remains to be seen. In the meantime Mildred & I have only
the clothes we stand in & they are none too cool; our nighties & tooth
brushes are with us thank fortune....

This ship is not quite so comfortable or nearly so large as the Asturias,
but there is nothing really to grumble at, & the meals are the best we have
had since leaving home. It seems very different, for the Stewards & sailors
on the other boat were all English, but here the Stewards are French-Indian
... & the sailors from India, black & Mohammedan. The latter wear supposedly white trousers, a blue shirt that comes to the knee, tied around the waist
with an old red bandana handkerchief, & on their heads a cross between the
red fez & turban.

The fighting in the Dardanelles as you no doubt have heard by now has
been very heavy, but suppose I mustn't enlarge on this, being a forbidden
subject.

... Saturday morning ... the O.C. wouldn't give anyone leave, & at 1 p.m. without a word we steamed out of the harbour, leaving the green water behind, & once again saw the wonderful blue sea of the Mediterranean. To-day (Sunday) we have occasionally had a glimpse of one of the many islands, rising in the distance, looking bare & barren, but just at sun-set a wonderful picture.

...

We expect to arrive in the morning (Monday Aug. 16th), & I am posting this immediately in the hopes it will go direct. Dear knows when we will get any mail. There are heaps of interesting things to tell you, but we are put on our honour regarding mentioning troops, & as our letters are censored by members of our own unit, think it wiser not to say too much about what I think of the various members.

...

Monday a.m. Aug. 16th

We are just at Lemnos but haven't reached the harbour yet – but must finish.

Heaps of love dear, & if you don't hear very regularly don't worry.

They say it is at least much cooler here – this is the only item on which *all* agree.

Always love
from Lollie.

2

Lemnos:
"Poor Souls" and "Pathetic Sights"

In 1915, the Allies attempted to capture the Dardanelles, "the narrow strip of water between Europe and Asia."[1] This catastrophic campaign was designed to force passage through to Russia and knock the Ottoman Empire out of the war.[2] When naval assaults on the Turkish forts in the Dardanelles failed in February and March, the War Council sent infantry to attack the steep, rocky heights of the Gallipoli Peninsula. The delay between the naval attack and the infantry landing, however, allowed the Turkish forces time to entrench on the peninsula's high ground. On April 25, 1915, British,[3] ANZAC,[4] and French troops attacked, only to be decimated in the landing boats and on the beaches by Turkish troops firing from the heights. Despite enormous casualties, the Allies established tenuous beachheads. Fighting continued under hellish conditions throughout the summer, with repeated Allied frontal assaults. Poor food, lack of water, dire heat, and a plague of flies led to widespread illness.[5]

Sir Ian Hamilton, the British commander of the Mediterranean Expeditionary Force, excluded medical officers from campaign planning. He also underestimated the number of casualties. This lack of foresight led to severe shortages of medical staff, transport for casualties, and equipment.[6] By June, "the medical services came near to breaking down."[7]

In France, transporting wounded and ill men was relatively systematic. In the Dardanelles, stretcher bearers had to carry soldiers down the rough, steeply pitched terrain to the beaches.[8] Mules were also used at times. The men came under fire on the journey and at the first aid posts on the beaches. Soldiers were then transported by lighters[9] to hospital ships and "black ships" for the journey to the nearest hospitals.[10] At first, men were shipped to Alexandria, Cairo, Malta, and England. Later, many were sent to hastily set up hospitals on the islands of Imbros and Lemnos. Many had not been examined or treated before leaving the beaches. Those on stretchers had to be winched onto the hospital ships.[11] Nurses and doctors on board worked flat out, dressing wounds and operating. The ships became a form of casualty clearing station.[12]

Repeated attacks in May and June meant a steady flow of wounded, but a plague of flies in June led to widespread dysentery and other enteric diseases. Up to one thousand ill men per week were being evacuated during the summer months.[13] Their inadequate diet of bully beef and jam and their limited supplies of water could not help them heal.[14]

The prolonged campaign and high casualty rates meant that better medical arrangements were badly needed. In July 1915, the British medical administration asked the Canadians for help. Three hospitals, CSHs Nos. 1, 3, and 5, were posted to the British MEF. Nos. 1 and 3 were sent to Lemnos, No. 5 to Cairo.[15] The two Canadian hospitals on Lemnos were among the first to include female nurses on their staffs.[16]

Laura and Mildred, with CSH No. 1, arrived on Lemnos in mid-August. For the next five months, Laura's and Mildred's letters vividly document the impact of the Gallipoli campaign and faulty British administration on the soldiers and the medical staff. It was a testing time for CSH No. 1. The unit had few medical supplies, poor equipment, scanty rations, and little water. When illness swept the staff, tensions within the unit became rife.

On August 22, CSH No. 1 received its first 309 patients, even though the unit was still erecting its tents.[17] Although the Allied attack on the Sari Bair ridge in August resulted in many severe casualties,[18] CSH No. 1 received mostly "acute enterics" and lightly wounded men.[19] In September, with many of its staff falling ill with diarrhea or dysentery, the hospital averaged 550 patients per day, a number that rose to over 600 in October, still primarily medical cases.[20] On November 27, the worst blizzard in "forty years" swept the peninsula and islands. Snow, rain, and sleet flooded the trenches, causing 10,000 casualties. Many soldiers drowned or froze to death.[21] On December 1, CSH No. 1 treated eight hundred soldiers for frostbite. Many suffered from frozen feet that required partial or entire amputation.[22]

The Allies abandoned the Gallipoli campaign and evacuated its soldiers from the peninsula in stages in December 1915 and January 1916. As Laura documents, the nurses joyously greeted the first evacuees from the peninsula in December. The last troops evacuated Cape Helles, at the southernmost tip of the peninsula, on the night of January 8–9, 1916.[23] Although the hospitals were prepared for casualties, miraculously, none occurred. With the campaign over, CSH No. 1 shut down on January 31, 1916.[24] Its medical staff did remarkable work under extreme conditions throughout their time there.[25]

Laura and Mildred were new to active service and knew few people in the unit. They were unprepared for a social hierarchy based on length of service and deftness in "recruiting supplies." They were equally unprepared for the real hardships of insufficient food and water. Yet the privations and illnesses the two suffered strengthened their friendship, and they tended to one another physically and emotionally. Laura's letters record growing tensions among the nurses and outright rebellion against the matron and other authorities. Competition and strife were even apparent at Christmas, when the nurses decorated the tents to boost patients' morale. Laura's letters also demonstrate her increasingly irritated reflections about gender roles and the place of professional nurses in wartime.

Laura's and Mildred's letters overturn public assumptions about war hospitals. They were not clean, comfortable places with well-fed soldiers and up-to-date equipment. The image of Mildred dispensing dysentery mixture from a used whiskey bottle instantly dispels such notions, as do the pair's determined efforts to obtain supplies to make their patients comfortable. Thrust from comfort into chaos and deprivation, the pair developed resilience and resistance through friendship and their professional skills. They justified their work and their presence in this "heart-breaking" place by reflecting that as nurses and as women they were doing their patients "some good."[26]

For the rest of Laura and Mildred's war, they remembered the hardships of Lemnos. No other posting, no matter how traumatic, would be as difficult to bear.

Letter No. 19
August 26th, 1915
No. 1 Canadian Stationary Hospital,
Lemnos

Dear Mother,

You have no idea how difficult it is at present to get a letter written, not that we are so terribly rushed, but we all more or less are feeling the climate, the days are very short, for once the sun goes down at 7 p.m. it is dark, & at present candle light is all we have in our tents, & things generally are in such a muddle, we just try to screw up enough energy to get a little wash & tumble into bed.[27]

...

Fortunately no patients arrived the 1st day, so we were able to get our things straightened out a little bit, but you can imagine with three in a tent (12 x 14 ft. open at both ends) & *all* our paraphernalia ... there isn't any too much room. There are only two poles, one at either end, so nowhere to put a nail of any sort. Fortunately they are lined with brown, so not so hot as the white.

The 1st day, meals were pretty bad, bully beef for breakfast & dinner, & jam for tea, but since have gradually improved, although they are nothing to boast of. I worse luck was un-fortunate enough to be made mess sister, & so responsible for all meals, which of course especially at the start is a rotten job, for you've only got what you're given, dishes at present are short, the stove four tins in the open ... [with] wood burning in the middle for the pots, & such like difficulties.

We have a man cook & his assistant & two men to help, but beyond the cook they all hate their work, & do just as little as they possibly can. Yesterday I managed to get some enamel ware, & rations were more plenti-ful. Unfortunately our one well of decent drinking water (it is a ¼ to ½ mile away, & there is about one horse to bring it all to camp, & the first two days it was carried in pails) has gone dry, & now we are forced to use another one in which the water is not good & so have to use chlorine, & it makes the tea taste like the devil – I'd give a £ for a good long cold drink.

Yesterday we had bacon & jam for breakfast 7.30 a.m. with tea – bread – no butter of course. What you can get about once a week is $1.25 a pound, & so rancid you can't eat it so decided we'd have to do without.

For lunch 12 noon. – hard boiled eggs with thickened milk, boiled rice & raisins – the latter rather soggy for in order to get enough done & so little room for pots, it's rather difficult to cook – of course chlorinated tea & cheese & jam, which are always in hand.

At 4 o'clock we have always afternoon tea. Yesterday made jam sandwiches, but the jam un-fortunately tasted of coal-oil in spite of the fact we haven't been able to get any yet, so they weren't awfully good.

... Then for dinner we had our daily portion of fresh beef, cooked semi-stew-pot-roast-fashion & a few potatoes, the first vegetable we have managed to get since coming, & they tasted more than good. We had a delicious melon ready for dessert, but an order came out in the afternoon that *no* melons on the Island were to be eaten, so per usual we fell back on jam! Boats are so very difficult to get, & so much in demand, we can't get out to the ships in the harbour in order to replenish our pantry a bit. Of course in time things will improve.

August 29th

Just here I was interrupted & have never since had a chance to sit down & finish but to-day my duties as Mess Sister ended.... It really has been an awful job especially at the start, for professionally our Matron is simply impossible. It's useless to go into details, but she is apparently the kind that's out for a good time, & while in some respects she is good to us in trying to get anything she can for our comforts, it is all spoilt by her unreasonableness & lack of control. To meet socially, if one didn't know her too well, she might be alright, but she is simply impossible to work with; fortunately at the start Mildred & I apparently made a good impression, so we have suffered rather less than others....

Well in spite of my troubles, the heat & the dirt, & general discomfort, I have had a wonderful week of it & feel that nothing will exceed my first impressions as regard interest.

The Hospital itself I will only just touch on, as I have, beyond walking through it, seen nothing of the work, all my time having been spent searching for food, getting it on the table in time, & trying to get the girls something to eat containing the fewest possible number of flies. To-day at dinner ... while eating, eight fell dead on my plate from over feeding, & I have become so hardened to the sight, I don't even pick them out & throw them on the floor but just keep a grave yard in one corner.

On the 27th the Quarter-master managed to get hold of a sail boat ... & ... the Padre, Miss Charleson (Matron), a Miss McC. ... & myself went off around the harbour in search of food. Taking me along was one of the many decent things the Matron has done.... We really had a great time, but didn't manage to get half we wanted, as we had to spend so much time trying to find out the Headquarters of the Red Cross here, we are so badly in need of surgical supplies. Wouldn't you think anyone coming here would be notified just where such a place would be? But no, endless time & money is spent finding out every little thing. Of course all this trouble in the Dardanelles was somewhat of a surprise, but the mis-management seems to be colossal. However I suppose it's easy to sit back & criticise – in France things run much more smoothly, but from all accounts *the* best men on the whole are there, & when a mistake is made, it can be so much more quickly rectified. Here it means weeks, if anything is forgotten, before it can be replaced.

On our 2nd day we got a number of patients & now have between four & five hundred. None of them very badly wounded, but a number of sick medical cases. Everyone agrees that the men from the Eastern front look much worse physically than the patients in France. Even those that are only slightly wounded look wrecks. The long summer of intense & continuous heat, combined with the bad food (bully beef & hardtack in a country where there is practically no water is a terrible diet) has taken all the life out of them, & they look terribly famished & exhausted....

Did I tell you the unit consisted of about 200 men (orderlies, etc.), 18 doctors, 26 nurses & a Matron? And we expect before long to be able to take 1000 patients. In the meantime we are not too rushed. So far there are no English Sisters on the island but the Australians have two General Hospitals, one with 80 nurses, but the other has none, only orderlies. Some of our girls the first three days went to the latter to help, & they said you only had to see a hospital run entirely by men to realize how much better things went where there are women ... particularly in regard to small comforts for the patients. Men too sick to drag their blankets off them, lying with two heavy blankets over them when it was over 100° [F] in the tent!!! And not an orderly thought of removing them – & such like details.

It is intensely interesting to watch a tent hospital grow, with patients coming & going at the same time, but the confusion is terrible. It is *that* & the looking for necessaries that tire the girls more than the actual work at present.

Mail arrived on the 26th ... the first in a month, & your letter ... amongst others. It was good to hear again, but when you answer regarding things we did in London it seems such ages ago!! Then the next day another mail arrived!! You can't imagine the excitement....

Have I ever told you we are now wearing Eton collars[28] with our working uniform – & when in Alexandria we were allowed to buy muslin ones. In fact we are allowed to wear much what we like, & already everyone has dispensed with cuffs. It's too hot for long sleeves, & laundry is frightfully expensive, to say nothing of being very badly done.

Mudros Harbour just at present is a wonderful sight, but we are not supposed to say much about it. We can't see it from the camp, except a small arm which runs in front for a short distance, merely looking like a pond, but although we are about two miles from any landing, it is not more than ten minutes walk from behind our tents to the water. However we can do no bathing – the out-let to the Harbour is so small that it doesn't give it a chance to get cleaned out when the tide changes, & consequently they say the water is a regular cesspool full of infection. You can imagine with numerous hospital ships, etc., what the refuse must be, not to mention the many who are buried there, for I feel sure none are brought on shore.

The kits of *all* the men going to the front are kept on this island, & the other day we passed the place where they are kept. You can imagine the sight;

thousands of course will never be claimed. It just made one feel sick to look at them.

Well, all these pages & not a word about the scenery. The day we came to the shore, the moon was just a few days old & the nights have been glorious. Generally quite a breeze, so for a few nights we didn't sleep very well, the tents flapping, & various un-usual noises waking us up constantly. From 5 p.m. until 9 a.m. the air is wonderful, & the outline of the mountains against the sun-set beyond description. But once that ever-lasting sun is well up over-head all the beauty for me is gone, & my day is spent in one-long-unspoken prayer that the evening will come quickly. The first few days were awful, but since then not quite so trying, & I've really stood it wonderfully well, far better than I anticipated.

We have had four or five nurses off sick ever since we came – all the same complaint; dysentery combined with nausea. So far I have escaped being on the sick list – had a very slight attack which I think in the end did me more good than harm. Most of the Officers have had their turn, & the majority of the men – so it seems inevitable. Can hardly expect to escape, but still have hopes.

Kastro, the capital of the island, several miles from here, ... is quite a large place, I believe 14,000 inhabitants. Thinking we might be able to get supplies there, & the Matron being rather keen on the outing, we got three mules yesterday & went in search of food.... Neither Miss Charleson or I ride, but were assured these mules were too starved & tired out to do any-thing un-expected, so we got on their backs, sitting side ways & having a loop of rope to use as a stirrup. One can hardly say they are comfortable in those primitive saddles, but ... one never feels nervous for a moment the animals are so sure of themselves; but we must have looked a picture. I wish I could give you an idea of the country. Frightfully barren – we went up hill & down hill, great barren rock, what might be grass after a rainy season, now like dried hay. Just outside the camp there are two small villages, & once past them, we didn't see a scrap of green for four miles, when we came on some sort of a vineyard, in the distance a most attractive looking spot, surrounded by a stone wall – but close to it didn't attract me.... Having passed this spot, we again went up & down rocky, barren, sandy mountains, the mules following the narrowest of foot paths, picking their way so dain-tily, going up the steepest inclines, nothing but sheer rock, & never making a false step.

Kastro itself is right on the sea with the most beautiful out-look. At the extreme end there is a steep rocky precipice, on the top of which is an old fort ... built about the 16th or 17th century, & partly destroyed in 1912 when

Greece took the place from Turkey; the ... old cannon balls are still scattered everywhere. It is now used as a look-out....

...

There is a square in the middle where apparently the whole population, (men of course, the women always seem to stay around the house), meet, sit around at tables & drink – drink – drink. No one does any work, & when you go in a shop to buy anything, the owner follows you in from somewhere in the street & serves you. There are very few Turks left on the island ... the whole population now being made up of Greeks.

...

Mildred is not looking very well – she has had the Gallipoli trot rather badly, or perhaps I should say quite continuously, but is somewhat better the past two days.

To-morrow I go to the Wards & expect as usual I shall hate it the first day, but after that it is much more interesting.

Well this time I'm really going to stop.... Am most anxious to hear what Temple is going to do.[29] I only hope if he comes across he will go to France & not here.

We're all covered with bites, but have stopped enquiring what kind & simply call them hives.[30]

Love to Uncle George & heaps for your own dear self from Lollie

Your letters are great....

Letter No. 20
Lemnos
September 1st, 1915

Dear Mother,

Two days ago I sent you a very lengthy epistle, & since then have been off sick with the common complaint, but fortunate in having it clear up so quickly. While it lasts it's awful! Cramps – back ache, pains in one's legs, a splitting headache & Temperature 102 [°F] on a day when it must have been 90 in the shade[31] & heaven only knows what in the sun, made me long for home & Mother, with a bath-room next door. As it was the constant runs to our W.C.[32] through the hot sun, yards & yards from our tent, about finished me. However I've recovered wonderfully quickly & while I'm spending the day in bed, expect to get busy again to-morrow.

The heat in our tent was simply un-bearable yesterday, but providence
sent a thunder-storm in the night with the result that to-day has been rather
dull, & comfortably cool, & once again I have hopes that the worst of the
heat is over & there are better things in store for us. Needless to say Mildred
has looked after me well, & been the greatest comfort.

Last night we had rather a scare. Our tents are on the outskirts of our
camp, & while from the front of the tent it is only a few yards to the
Officers' Quarters, at the back we look out on a wide expanse of barren
ground, ending in a ridge. Across this expanse one quite often sees a ... man
(there are various men around – Arabs – Hindus, etc.) wander, in his rags &
poverty.... [T]hey are fearful looking creatures & when one happens to
think of them at night, it's all up. Of course our tents have to be kept wide
open to get what little breeze happens to be around – & last night there was
quite a gale blowing – that, combined with rather a severe thunder-storm,
our tents flapping to beat three of a kind, meant we were all awake. On
glancing outside, we saw what appeared to be a straight line of black objects
advancing [with] not a sound to be heard, although [they] came nearer &
nearer. Our hearts were in our mouths, when one yard nearer seemed to
bring them within proper range & we realized ... the line was only an immense herd of sheep!!

Once again we settled down to sleep, having just driven the beasts back,
when Galt decided to fasten one side of the tent & saw someone standing
outside. Thinking it might be one of the girls, called out, & on receiving no
answer, gave a yell, Mildred simultaneously had night-mare & woke with an
awful scream – by this time I was sitting up in bed silent but scared green.
Then we realized the silent figure was a poor soul from the next tent so sick
she couldn't speak for a moment – by this time we were *all* laughing so hard
we almost went into hysterics. Every night something unforeseen happens,
and it was a great relief this morning when Major Williams informed us a
fence was to be put up at the back. There are of course several guards on
duty at night, but so far apart, anyone might get through. However, imagine
there is no need for anyone to worry, but either the climate or the East
generally seems to have got everyone's nerves on end.
...

... I had just one day in the Wards & like the work immensely. It certainly is quite different from anything I have experienced before. In one
sense a nurse can do so little beyond medicines & Temperatures & dressings, especially here where there is no water to wash them with, at least so
far there hasn't been enough. Will tell you more about the work in my next.

Au revoir for the present – my letter may sound rather grumbly but we're really alright & every day things are improving.

Poor Colonel McKee has been about the sickest of the lot. In fact the officers as a whole have been worse I think than we have.

Will write soon again but don't worry if you don't hear, for the mails we are told are frightfully un-certain.

Love to Uncle & Temple when you write for I feel sure he must have left by the time you receive this.

Heaps of love to your own self from Yours lovingly
Lollie.

P.S. It has suddenly occurred to me in your last letter but one, you asked one or two questions regarding our mess uniforms.... The reason we generally wore our capes even on warm days was that they hid our buttons & stars,[33] & no one specially noticed us, but without them all sorts & conditions of men passed remarks as we went by, others felt privileged to stop & more or less try to "pick us up," while others just politely inquired who we were. But "everyone" considered they had a right to talk to us as we were in uniforms....

Letter No. 21
Lemnos
September 6th, 1915

Dear Mother,

...

First & foremost I'm feeling heaps better, & we've had, in spite of the usual persistent sun-shine to-day, a fairly cool breeze & rather fewer flies, so feel "things are looking up."

Meals are still pretty bad for ourselves, largely owing to our Matron, who seems to antagonize everyone with whom she comes in contact. They would be pretty bad anyway, for no one has made any provision for the newcomers, in fact rather the reverse, & we won't have proper food until we send either to Alexandria or England, & of course where there are so few boats & so much is needed, this means time. The bread, which is made on the Island by the Government (English) ..., has been so sour, the medical men ... have forbidden us to eat it. This means we have had only hard-tack for a week, & as vegetables are very scarce, either canned or otherwise, meat is our main-stay, a mighty poor diet for this climate.

...

I simply can't put all the circumstances down on paper – it's too long a tale – one doesn't mind what can't be helped, but when it's a case like the present it makes one mad.

And after this trip I'll never believe it's only the *Canadian* Government that has flaws in it – for the management of this end of affairs makes one sick at heart. We can only hope the out-look is not quite so bad as it appears on the surface. I'm not so pessimistic yet that I think we won't win out in the end, but I haven't a doubt that the sacrifice through ignorance & incapability of many of the heads has been much worse than necessary. It is dreadful to hear the men talk about it; they simply feel they are being slaughtered, & I'm afraid it's only too true. And then how they suffered in this devilish climate!

To-day Sir Ian Hamilton inspected the Camp,[34] but as I was not on duty at the time, did not see him, & am afraid wasn't interested enough to bother very much – it was too hot! But he is no hero to the men back from the front. No doubt they judge him un-fairly, but evidently his personality doesn't please the Tommie.

Well to get on a slightly more cheerful strain—

The men's food in the Line (Ward is *not* the proper term in a Tent Hospital) has certainly improved, although of course they are suffering from the lack of bread also – but the canned milk is better than it was, not so sickeningly sweet, & there is canned soup for those on fluids, although none for our Mess.

The scarcity of water still continues, & I think the flies are even worse than before, certainly more stupid, & in greater number.

Well here I am at it again, but don't imagine for one minute I have a regret in coming – for now I am working in the hospital I love it, hot & dirty as it is. Fleas I no longer give a thought to, my meals I eat off dishes covered with fly marks without a thought, & gaze at "live stock"[35] on the men without a qualm!

The patients are wonderfully good – you never hear a grumble except from those who have been in hospitals a long time; it's marvelous how they stand pain. I am a little disappointed we don't get the *bad* cases, for only those who they have hopes of recovering sufficiently to return to the lines come here.

...

...[O]ne of the naval officers came & invited any of the nurses over for afternoon tea that could go.... Hadn't the slightest inclination to go, for hadn't had a bite to eat for three days except about two sweet biscuits, but couldn't work, & as Mildred was another of the number, that decided me, & it did me heaps of good.

A motor lorry happened to be in the camp, having brought up supplies, so we commandeered it to take us down to the wharf, ... [where] we were met by a small launch, which took us to the boat. It is stationed here as a supply boat, & ... they gave us a dandy meal, & ... more to take home! ...

In a conversation with the Principal Medical Officer, the first man I met, we got on the subject somehow of the lack of water, & before I realized it had suggested a bath, which he promptly took up – & on the q.t. I rushed down to his bath-room where he had made the necessary arrangements, & with Mildred to protect me, had my first experience of an English tin-bath. You can picture me sitting in this little tin affair, at an afternoon tea party!!! I never even stopped to take my hat off.

You can imagine the condition of affairs when I tell you Mildred insisted on getting in after me!

The whole incident only took up ten minutes of our precious time. Of course the grub was the main feature of the affair, & little scraps of news we obtained. Also some of the Australian Sisters were there, such nice girls. The men were only so-so & there were so many of us, the conversation ... was general.

On the way home at 9 p.m. when we were passing the Scottish Convalescent & Clearing Hospital, some of the officers came out & accosted us & gave us an invite to go & listen to a concert they were having for the men in the open.... There must have been several hundred patients sitting around in a circle, the stage being in the middle, & marvellous to relate, there was a piano – an awful thing, but it sounded mighty good to us. Afterward we had a cup of tea & some sandwiches & came home about 9.30 p.m.

...

Poor Mildred the last few days has been nearly eaten alive – by what we're not sure. So far we have caught nothing worse than fleas, though some of the other girls have been less fortunate.

I read very little, for I find the glare of the sun pretty trying & have to rest my eyes when the sun is up as much as possible – & at night it's almost impossible. Had I known what it is like would have invested in a good light. In the Lines they have an acetylene light, which is fine.

Colonel McKee has been awfully ill since arriving, & his medical advisor is trying to persuade him to go back to England for a few months rest – so far however he has refused. He had a bad attack of dysentery, & doesn't seem able to throw it off.

Well good bye for the present. Don't worry about us, for each week they say the weather improves, & we may be moved any time, the life is so uncertain, or we may stay here a year.

Love to Uncle George & Temple. So far haven't been able to get any letters written except to yourself & one or two to England to let them know we had arrived.

Am wondering when the next mail will arrive. Always love to you as ever from
Lollie

Lemnos
September 7th, 1915

My dear Cairine,

It was so nice to find a letter from you amongst the first mail we received. Our letters come very irregularly, sometimes twice a week, & perhaps not again for ten days. I hope the day never arrives that there are no letters for me, for we just live for mail.

Well Rockland seems in another world[36] – & I really wonder when I will see you all again. Things seem so tied up at this end that I am afraid it will be a long time before we get home.

We have had terribly uphill work here – no one knows the hardships we have put up with. Imagine planting a hospital on a desert island! for it is practically that. With the exception of a few little Greek villages, filthy dirty & very primitive, there is nothing here. The island is quite large – about twenty miles long – & once the sun sets it looks attractive. It is rather hilly, but not *one* tree or a blade of grass. Just sand & rocks – a few thistles. The sun is awful – I never felt such *intense* heat – & the flies!!! I cannot describe them. Luckily the evenings are cool, so we get our sleep in peace.

Water is very scarce. All we use is carted from a well which is ¼ of a mile away. It runs dry often, then they send the Mule teams off for miles in search of water. It is not fit for us to drink – & we get a *very* small allowance for washing.

Our tents are splendid. We have the square ones made by your friends "Smart-Woods." They are very roomy – 14 ft. square. Three of us are in a tent. Cecily Galt, Lollie & I are all together. It is "active service" with a vengeance.

Of course we have been about starved since our arrival. It seems customary for the English Government to send a Hospital Unit to a desert island, & make *absolutely* no provision for them. This is true & no exaggeration. I think when everything is over an inquiry will be made into the way things have been mismanaged out East.

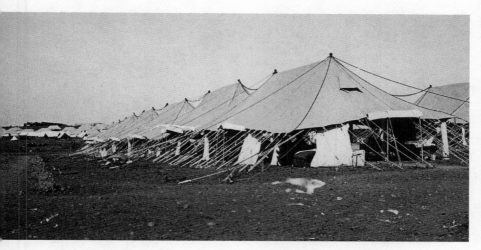

A hospital ward, Mudros. *George Metcalf Archival Collection, Canadian War Museum. CWM 20070103-015_p21a*

We could not draw food – & now that we are getting it, it is fit for Esquimaux – so you can imagine in a tropical climate what it is like. In consequence, we have all been ill in turn. The trouble is the climate & conditions are such that once one gets ill, it is so hard to pick up. The bread made by the Army Service Corps has been so bad that we have all had hard tack for five days. No fresh vegetables are to be had, no butter, no fruit – practically nothing but tough meat, bully beef & jam. You would think that with Alexandria just two days from here that a supply ship might come along to us with stuff.

You will think I am a fearful grumbler – but these are facts.

The patients started coming in the day after we arrived. None of them have been very bad cases. I have an idea they will just send us the ones who will be able to return in a short time. We have about 450 at the present.

I am in a Medical "line" which holds 92 patients. Mostly all the cases are dysentery. They all say conditions are awful where they come from – wrong food, & so little water. They only get it every other day. One man told me that when his comrade was dying beside him he was not *allowed* to give him a drink of water, for it has to be kept for the well people who will live. Doesn't it seem awful?

We can give so little to the men, for we have so few things to work with. The girls say in France they were surfeited with necessities & comforts – here we can get practically nothing for the Men. Fancy no nightshirts for them.

Twenty-seven new patients arrived tonight in the line I am in. I only had six *flannel shirts* to give them for nightshirts! It seems terrible when you think there is such a supply being made. I think the reason is the people in authority thought this was to be such a short piece of work that it was not worthwhile bothering.

... There are quite a few camp Hospitals here, two Australian, two Canadian (including ourselves) & a couple of R.A.M.C. ones, all in various stages of despair!!

...

My letter looks very crumpled – please excuse it – and with much love to all.

Affectionately yours.
Mildred H. Forbes

Lemnos
Letter No. 22
September 16th–20th, 1915

Dear Mother,

...

Yesterday was indeed a Jonah day for both Mildred & myself.... [W]e went on duty Sunday for night work, & owing to flies, light & noise, slept but little Monday & Tuesday, [so] felt more than abused that our third day should have been such as it was.

To begin with about 5.30 a.m. Mildred, who also is on night duty, rushed in to tell me ... to go & look at the sun-[rise], & it certainly was one of the most beautiful sights I have ever seen. Half the sky was covered with soft, fleecy clouds, all various shades of pink, rose & soft purples, while just near the horizon, the softest yellow coloring. It was wonderful.

When we came off duty, were told that owing to the Colonel being able to let us have three extra tents, in future it would be possible to have just two nurses in a tent, so as Galt was willing to move, decided that ... we would get a man to take her things to another tent, & so get settled a bit. This meant it was 11 a.m. before we got to bed; by this time clouds had gathered, the wind had risen, & it began to rain, when I heard someone outside saying *mail* had arrived, the first for about ten days! So jumped out of bed & put on my sou-wester & waterproof & rushed over to the Matron's office, & was terribly disappointed to find there was no letter from you.... This was blow no. 1.

Came back to bed, & previous to getting in decided to examine my
clothes, as I had received several bites during the night, & to my disgust
(they no longer fill me with horror) found a member of the livestock family
– this is getting to be a daily occurrence!! Imagine what a fit one would take
over such an experience at home, while here, beyond the discomfort, one
takes it as a matter of no consequence!!!

Finally we settled down to sleep feeling pretty tired, for we hadn't had more
than three hours sleep daily for three days, when suddenly a hurricane began
to blow, the heavens poured forth her wrath, & before you could say "scat!"
a river two inches deep ran through our tent from one side to the other, & I
thought our tent would fall down on our heads. Fortunately my rubber boots
were beside my bed, so jumped out quickly, pinned up my nightie, & proceeded to gather up boots, hold-alls, etc., & piled them up on my trunk, then
got back into bed, feeling I had done all I could & would have to trust to
luck regarding the rest. By 2 o'clock the rain had ceased, but the storm had
done no end of damage, & they immediately got out a squad of men to dig
trenches & drain off the water, some to tighten up ropes of tents, etc. This
occasioned endless shouting of orders, which meant we got about an hour's
sleep in all, & when it came time to dress for dinner, we left our beds feeling
life was somewhat hopeless. I simply can't describe the wetness of everything,
& the *mud* – the latter could only be appreciated by the pioneers of Winnipeg.[37] It's the kind that sticks & piles up on the soles of one's boots until they
are so heavy one feels water-logged. My canvas dunnage bag ... was soaked
through; the one bright spot was when I opened my trunk, & found it had
stood the test of standing in three inches of water & remaining perfectly dry!

As it began to rain again ... we pinned up our skirts turkish fashion, [&]
wore our waterproofs, sou-westers & rubber boots on duty. I can't begin to
describe the "Line." Fortunately they had been able, by moving beds, to
keep them all dry, but the floors were something awful. Owing to receiving
patients almost before the tents were up, they couldn't take time to level the
ground, & so the tarpaulin was laid on very un-even rocky ground, with the
result that after such a storm, the hollows held ... four & five inches of water
... quite comfortably, & every bit ... a mass of slippery clay-like mud. Many
a time I nearly landed on my head! What with the wind, my three smoky
lanterns, & one patient at death's door all night, it was quite spooky. So
many of the men from the front have a habit of talking or calling out loud
in their sleep that at times it is rather startling, though I must say I seldom
feel nervous, for most of the time there is an orderly in the tent. But a line
containing 55 beds on either side is quite a length. My sick patient, such a
nice Irish boy, died to-day at noon & we all feel very badly.

To-night everyone is very quiet & for the past two hours I have practically had nothing to do. The work changes so from day to day. Yesterday 25 quite sick patients left our Line for England, & while their beds are again filled, their places have been taken by medical patients, so having no dressings, the work is much lighter.

There is no wind at all to-night & every now & again the stillness is broken by the sound of the bombarding up at the Peninsula, faint but un-mistakable. Of course many of the boats only take three hours to get there from here.

There is just the wildest possibility we may in time be sent to the Island of Imbros, which is within 20 miles ... of the front, & am rather keen to go, for we couldn't have more to put up with there than we have had here, & the work would be much more interesting. However probably nothing will come of it.

Mildred has been feeling very miserable this week. Night duty never agrees with her, & she cannot get rid of what is known in our own country as "summer complaint."[38] I really am quite worried about her, & have finally persuaded her to come off duty in the morning for a day or two, for nothing helps to clear up this trouble so quickly as complete rest. Thank goodness beyond my three days of it I have practically been free of it, & now that the weather is so much cooler, am feeling fine & eating well.

No. 3 Canadian Stationary Hospital, ... next to ours, have suffered very much more than we have. The Colonel ... has been miserable ever since putting his foot on the island, & is now laid up. The Matron as soon as she is well enough to stand the trip is to be invalided home; three nurses & two doctors *were* invalided home this week – & of course one of their nurses died, as I told you before.[39]

Just at present our own Matron is ill, & one of our nurses who could not get over her attack has been sent back to England. Otherwise all the "Sisters" have more or less recovered from their attacks. Colonel McKee has had an awful time of it. Beyond the first week has been in bed all the time, & rumour says he will have to be invalided home for good, as he has one of the severe types of dysentery that cannot be cured in this climate....

...

... Each day seems to bring its own difficulty. To-day we had orders that *all* drinking water had to be boiled. You can imagine keeping 110 men supplied with drinks, when we have only three small primer stoves (coal-oil) with one burner on each to boil the water on, for the kitchen has all it can do to manage the meals. Consequently no one has had enough, & it follows there is a feeling of discontent in the atmosphere. To-night the coal-oil gave out as no one on the island possesses any, so we are worse off than ever. Our Orderly has just been over & started the fire going in the kitchen to boil a little for the morning.

The water supply is managed entirely by the British Director ... of Medical Services, & he is responsible for all these orders & likewise the lack of coal oil – each day something seems to be lost. To-morrow we hope to have stoves – at least they have been promised; imagine the amount of wood it will take to keep them all going. [N]o coal seems to be amongst the head-quarters supplies, & when one realizes all the wood has to be brought off the ships, you can see what an undertaking it all is.

There has been no fresh meat for four days, but as we managed to buy some curry off one of the boats, bully beef flavored with this & boiled rice makes a mighty good meal.

...

One of the officers went off on a shopping expedition the other day, so gave him 5 £ to get what he could.[40] He came back with a case of oranges, another of apples, a box of biscuits & a case of ginger ale, so sold some to the other girls & we have all been having a treat.

The men go round to the various boats in the harbour, tell a tale of woe, & try to persuade them to sell us something. Sometimes we get it & some-times we don't! It's rather humiliating to think this is necessary, when one knows in France the government supplies a Canteen almost everywhere. Here we have a small one where they charge exorbitant prices, are sold out every other day, & practically keep nothing.

...

September 19th, evening

...

Yesterday finally Mildred consented to come off duty, & really is feeling miserable but think now she has consented to lay up, the trouble will clear up quickly, for she has none of the more serious symptoms – but continuous diarrhoea is frightfully weakening. Mildred is not mentioning this last attack to her family, so should you see any of them, don't enlarge on the subject.

I came off night duty this morning & am awfully glad. I like the night work immensely but as we are situated, it is absolutely impossible to get any sleep, so noisy, the tents so light, & around noon ... the sun seems to con-centrate on one's tent, & it's always hot. However you can stand anything for a week, & while I didn't get more than two hours sleep to-day, spent the day in bed & ... to-night will get a good rest.

This coming week we expect to get the hospital moved into wooden huts, if another unit doesn't arrive to take possession before we get in, but think we may have to wait some time before they get accommodations for the unit. However the huts are about as close to our sleeping tents as the Tent Lines are....

Some of the girls went off on one of the boats in the harbour to a luncheon party, & came back with quite a supply of food, including 17 tins of butter – so we will have a treat to-morrow. Our first since landing! I was invited but altogether too tired to go.

Well it's late so must go to bed. Oh! forgot the most important thing of all. A mail came in yesterday & brought your letter....

...

We seem to get so little news away out here, either personal or otherwise, but live on rumours.... Love to Uncle Geo. & your own dear self.

As ever, Lollie.

[P.S.] ...

Lemnos
September 25th, 1915

Dear Mother,

...

Well dear I am afraid you may start & worry when you read in the paper, as you probably will, that the Matron of No. 3 Hospital has died – this is the second from that Unit & several others, as I told you, were invalided home, & there are others to follow. Of course it has cast a gloom over everything, & to the out-sider seems curious that one unit should have suffered from the effects of the country so much more than another. No doubt it is partly coincidence, & we hear that from a sanitary point of view, their camp can't be compared with ours – also their unit has seen but little of active service in comparison, & consequently [is] less able to cope with difficulties that arise.[41]

I wouldn't even mention this outside, because it doesn't do to repeat anything of this kind – but do feel there is little for you to worry over as regards conditions in our Camp. [C]onsequently un-less the unforeseen happens, [there is] no reason why we shouldn't be perfectly healthy in our work, especially now that we have ... a committee in our Mess & have been able to procure some food off the boats in port. Later on we may not be able

to continue doing so, if the much talked of gales blow with the force they
are credited with, but there is no use crossing this bridge until we come to it,
& by that time we may be far off from here.

In the meantime our meals are A.1. & Miss Upton using all her energy
& ingenuity to make the food appetizing & plentiful, & so far is succeeding
wonderfully. Her first day in charge we had beef-steak (tough but good),
fried onions & scalloped potatoes, ending up with a mighty good bread
pudding. My appetite is huge, one even a Navvie[42] would be proud of.

Mildred is still in bed, & sick to death of the monotony of life. To-day
she has "another trouble" to add to her misery, but hopes once this is past
to be able to get up once again. In writing to her family has scarcely mentioned being "off color," so don't you.

...

I was rather glad I could not get off duty to-day to go to the funeral, for
we couldn't all go, & it does up-set me. It's simply terrible – the loneliness
of it all! Imagine how all the nurses of that Unit must feel – for Mrs. Jaggard
seems to have been liked immensely personally, & since being on the Island,
has been indefatigable in her attentions to the nurses "off sick," & couldn't
do enough for the poor girl who died. Dysentery was the trouble, & of
course she wasn't a young woman.

In spite of having some time off each day, couldn't manage to get a few
lines off to you yesterday, for our tent was so un-tidy had to turn to & make
it a little more presentable for the "sick patient," & at night with the wind
blowing & only a poor lone flickering candle for light, gave up in despair
& went to bed.

To-day has been a nightmare from start to finish. It was decided all in a
hurry to move the whole hospital over to the [huts] – & never have I seen
such mis-management – or perhaps I should say apparent mis-management.
I simply can't describe the chaos – & heaven only knows what will happen
to-morrow, we left everything in such a muddle. So many things went
wrong – men detailed from other camps to come & help didn't turn up, etc.
... The huts are only half finished, there are Egyptians working all around
outside, the distances are immense, & altogether long to be back in our nice
old Indian Tents. On the other hand, although they may be draughty, &
you can see daylight between each board, at least there are floors – so easy to
walk on, & imagine when the rain comes down, while there may be a few
leaks, the floors won't be covered with water.

Perhaps in a day or so I'll be writing that everything is lovely.

We are still living in Tents & probably will for some time.

...

Well dear, thanks to the wind dying down for a few days, our candle has given a better light than last night, but it has burnt down, & is pretty late so had better say good-night....

Heaps of love dear, & I do hope you aren't worrying over me.

Love to all, Yours lovingly
      Lollie.

Letter No. 24
Lemnos
October 1st, 1915

Dear Mother,

...

Mildred is still in bed but feeling much more like her own self, although even yet she has not entirely got rid of that persistent diarrhoea. However Major Williams[43] has just been in & given her permission to get up to-morrow for a little while, so hope now she is really on the mend.

We are looking forward once she is up & around to get[ting] away from our own Camp for a few hours, & ... explor[ing] some of the surrounding villages. It is now over three weeks that I have been anywhere outside my own tent & my own special Line. [I]t makes life a little monotonous but it has been simply desperate for Mildred, shut up in a tent day after day, & [I] felt I wanted to spend all the time possible with her – & at the best it hasn't been much, for we have been very busy since the move. One wonders if things will ever straighten, for as soon as they do – then something happens, causing the same trouble all over again. Of course moving into the Huts when they are only half finished has made it much more difficult. [T]hen at present we only have accommodation for 350 patients & I believe we have 475, so it means a shortage of everything. However no doubt things will straighten out before long – in the meantime there is more or less confusion, everyone is over worked, the place is not ... kept up to the usual standard, consequently criticism is the order of the day & everyone feels a little peevish & nerves more or less on edge. I worry less & less every day, which is a good thing for my health if not for my conscience. But it is heart-breaking to be able to do so little for the men – the shortage is appalling. To-night no eggs in the Camp, so the patients had none for tea, & as the majority are allowed *no* bread owing to its being such a fearful dough, it means they get a watery cup of tea, & arrow-root made with water & a little canned milk for their evening meal. Pretty hard lines for men some of whom have been months at the front, living on nothing but bully beef & jam & even that sometimes bad! If they see cigarettes once a week here they are lucky – & what is worse we can't even *buy* stuff if we had the money.

Another shortage is coal-oil, consequently we are reduced to candles! This means from 6 p.m. the men can't see to do anything, for three candles to 45 beds doesn't give much illumination. To-night for the first time in ten days we have one coal-oil lantern to a hut & one or two candles!!

These are only a *few* of the many difficulties that arise daily & make our work so dis-heartening; the majority of them difficulties that were never encountered in France – that seems to have been a land of plenty. We simply long for a Canadian Red Cross branch in the East. Don't you think you could, with the assistance of Mrs. Kerry, induce your Chapter[44] to interest themselves in our Hospitals here?

The Canadian Hospitals in France seem to have made a wonderful name for themselves in France, from the patients' point of [view], & English, Scotch & Irish alike clamour to get into one in preference to their own. [B]ut [I] am afraid we are not making any such impression here, although patients who have left to go to the convalescent Camp near[by] come back with tales of how much better off they were with us.

I was talking with such a nice Englishman to-night who told me he had been at the Peninsula for five months, & for the past three had *never* been out of the trenches once, but had been on duty two hours & off two hours night & day for all that time – then he comes here with pleurisy, & we can give him *so little*. Do you wonder we feel there is mis-management somewhere?

Of course I know you would never print anything I write, but be careful about reading some of these things to outsiders, for I wouldn't like a lot that I tell you to be talked of outside as coming from this Camp.

...

Well dear, it is pretty late so won't give any details regarding the huts to-night. There seems so much to tell, & it takes such a long time to put on paper in spite of my pen rushing ahead, & never stopping to think. Mildred sends love & a whole heap always

      from Lollie.

P.S. Can't remember whether I told you what the men needed most in any of my letters, in case some of your friends think of sending anything.

Cigarettes & *Pipes*
Khaki handkerchiefs (they love to take them back to the front if they go.)
Shaving soap
Biscuits
Chocolate or sweets of any kind
Playing cards
In fact I might say almost any thing

Once again au revoir.
            Lollie.

[P.S.] ...

                                                                    Lemnos
                                                            October 1st, 1915

My dear Cairine,

...

Was so glad to hear you were all enjoying St. Andrews[45]....

You are so up in history that I wish you in your next would send me a few items about Lemnos – I am so ignorant, & declared that the only time I ever heard of it was when St. Paul visited it. Upon searching The Acts I can find no mention of the fact!!

We had about a week's respite from the heat – but today we have a very hot sticky day & innumerable flies. However there is promise of a cooler season, which keeps us alive.

Conditions are improving here in some respects. We are managing to get a little more food, shopping from the various ships that are in Mudros Harbour, so it means we are getting a supply of canned goods. The bread continues to be very bad. I wish the A.S.C. could be taught how to make it.

The patients have been moved into their new winter quarters, i.e. wooden huts. Thirty-five beds in a hut. After the tents they seem stuffy, but when the rain & gales come on we will appreciate some kind of shelter. Our huts will be ready for us shortly; in the meantime we like our tents very much, in spite of the centipedes & scorpions which are about. I say I shall return either very brave, or a nervous wreck. I fear the latter.

Don't think I am seeing ghastly sights, for we are not. Most of our cases are medical – very little surgery comes to us. In many respects it is a good thing, for this is a bad climate for wounds to heal & we cannot give the patients proper food. Being a stationary Hospital we don't keep long cases –

we rarely have a patient over two weeks. Typhoids are sent to the Australian General Hospital on this Island, then cases who are not gaining but who will be fit for duty in a month we transfer to Alexandria, others to England. So we have a shifting population. 200 will go out & before we can get the beds made, new ones turn up.

Although we don't see horrors, we are hearing of & seeing pathetic sights all the time, & it is heart-breaking not to have food to give the poor souls. Never at any time was the food plentiful or good, & now it is being cut down. At the head of affairs there is very bad work being done. I think the person ordering supplies for the Island has absolutely no idea of proportion. I believe there are several supply ships in, but in loading them they carefully put the food in the bottom, & then piled lumber & odds & ends on top which it will take some time to remove. That is a sample of the way things are done.

It seems a shame to think of so much going to the troops in France. They are inundated there with comforts of all kinds. People say they have more than they can use – yet we get so little for the men here. The British Red Cross are supposed to look after us, but it is more neglect than anything else. The men have not had cigarettes or pipes for over a week.

We (Lollie & I) have written to England for cigarettes, shaving soap & khaki handkerchiefs for the men. So far our parcels have arrived safely, so we thought we would get in a supply to give to our favorites.

It is strange we get so little news of what is going on at the Peninsula. The men cannot tell us, for they are working more or less in the dark.

We did hear of the good news from France. I know everyone longs for peace – but it seems out here, we just live for it.

With all our varied and trying experiences I would not leave if I got the chance tomorrow, for I feel we are doing some good. We heard some of the tales told by men who had been in one of the Hospitals here without nurses, & it was awful to hear what the poor creatures had to go through.

The British have only recently sent their Sisters here. I suppose by sending Australian & Canadian ones they would see how they stood it – before venturing to send their own. But we will show them ... the stuff we are made of.

...

> With Much love to you all.
> Affectionately yrs.
>   Mildred H. Forbes

Letter No. 25
Lemnos
October 8th, 1915

Dear Mother,

... There are one or two Officers who will censor our letters for us personally without reading them & naturally we prefer this to having them remain
open for the public-censors, consequently frequently have to let a day or so
pass before we can get the right man at the right moment, & as I have been
in bed since Monday, have had to let someone else do this work for me. I don't
know just what the trouble has been, *not* diarrhoea, but some slight infection,
causing headache, backache, & a small Temp. [B]eyond feeling absolutely
rotten however it is nothing serious. To-day my headache left me & with it
the Temp., so expect to be up again to-morrow. Many of the girls have had
it & Major Williams seems to think it is caused by the sudden return of the
heat, etc. etc. Too long a tale to go in to when there are more interesting
things to write about. It comes quickly & leaves one the same way.

Well I think it was last Saturday I sent you my last. We had three awfully
hot & terribly busy days. Sunday night I came off with my head just splitting, a touch of diarrhoea etc., so was told to stay off on Monday, & haven't
... been back on duty since. It's been mighty nice having Mildred here with
me in the tent, for naturally where nurses are so scarce, & our Matron *such*
a woman, one isn't over-showered with attention.

Mildred is not mentioning anything to her family at all about feeling or
rather having been sick, for she is feeling much better, has been up & around
the tent the past two days, is to get dressed this afternoon, & I do hope her
troubles are over. But the diarrhoea (*not* dysentery) has been so persistent,
Major Williams says she must be careful & go slowly. Imagine it will be three
weeks to-morrow since she went to bed! I shall be so thankful when we both
have the time & energy to go for a walk beyond the hospital lines, for it is
now five weeks since we have been outside our tent or Ward, & one is apt to
get a little hipped, especially where in one sense our work is so depressing &
un-satisfactory.

The men *are* so ill & so miserable, we have such a scarcity of not only
supplies but orderlies & nurses, that it makes work most difficult; & yet
when one stops & thinks about it we really are one & all very happy in our
work, & it is a satisfaction in knowing how much worse off they would be
without us. But how they all poor souls long for England, or some land
where food is plentiful & not *all* canned, where the sun is less penetrating,
& water less of a luxury.

Mrs. McKee has arrived at last, in full uniform & with the rank of a C.A.M.C. nurse, & with her Mrs Casgrain, wife of the Colonel of No. 3 Canadian Stationary Hospital; needless to say it makes us all mad to think of any un-professional being given the same rank,[46] for it certainly is not fair, although we all realize in this instance it was a means to an end – but if ever anyone had suffered for breaking regularities they have. Mrs. Casgrain arrived to find that her husband had left the same day for England, with but small chance of living until he reached there. She is still here, waiting to get *"invalided"* home, which is taking some time – but it is the only way it can be managed.

...

Major Williams came in the afternoon to see us both, & I begged to get up to-day, but he insisted on both of us staying in bed for one more day, so you see we have a cautious man looking after us. I really think he is wise, for of course all our work is amongst dysentery patients & so much depends on one feeling in good condition, & know he won't let us start in too soon.

...

Oct. 11th, morning

Another day of bright sun-shine, am up, dressed & feeling much more like my own self.

Mildred has just written to her sister & tells me she mentioned having been sick but that it was all over, so it doesn't matter now what you say.

I don't think I have ever told you we frequently, when the wind is in the right direction, can hear the big guns up at the front, & occasionally hear a few go off in the night much nearer – these must be more or less chance ones. It is surprising how near those at the front sound sometimes.

...

If you could get just one glimpse at my hair I know I would have your sympathy. It is straight as can be, oily & filthy in every way, & yet I dread more than words can tell the thought of washing it. I believe before long the Sisters are to be allowed a Sawyer stove for their own use. They are just a large round affair, in the lower part of which wood or fuel can be burnt, & the upper part is a huge sort of bowl arrangement for water. The thought of having warm water to wash in at night is indeed a luxury.[47]

Well dear ... I seem to have written such volumes about so little. I often wonder if in the end you get really any *idea* of what the place & work actually is – I *don't think* it would be possible to exaggerate it.

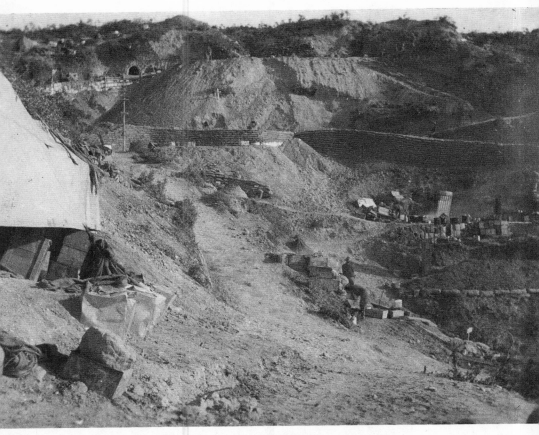

Cape Helles, Gallipoli Peninsula. *George Metcalf Archival Collection,*
Canadian War Museum. CWM 19790413-012-p20b

Good-bye once again. Love to Uncle. I can quite understand it must be
a relief to him to have Temple really off instead of waiting & wondering
when his commission would come. No matter what happens the boy will
be happier for having done what he has, but of course if he is one of the
un-fortunates, Uncle will be the one to suffer. But if only one could be out
here & see the type they are sending back, supposedly well, one can't help
but feel the healthier ones at home should be taking their place.

...

Good-bye & always love to you dear
       from Lollie.

Lemnos
October 22nd, 1915

My dear Cairine,

It is difficult to realize that we were suffering with the heat a short time ago, for tonight we are shivering in our huts. There is a strong wind blowing, raining, and the cracks in our huts so large that the draught almost blows me off my chair! The temperature is about what we get in the latter part of November at home. It certainly is a country of changes.

I think last time I wrote you we were in our tents. Since then much has happened. At the time of writing I was off duty sick – I don't believe I mentioned it for I did not want to have people anxious – so decided to wait till I was better before telling. They kept me in bed for three weeks. I was not so very ill, but had the usual complaint of this country. However I am well again & at work.

One night a few weeks ago – Miss Holland was ill in bed at the time & I was up for the first time – we had a fearful storm. Torrents of rain, thunder & lightning & finally a sort of cyclone – which brought our tent down over our heads! Never shall I forget the experience. The sensations I felt trying to get Lollie safely out of bed, & seeing all our belongings thrown on the wet & muddy ground from off the packing case which constituted our dressing table. We were two pitiful objects staggering out into the dark stormy night, leaving our "home" in what seemed to be ruins. That night eight of us (all in the same homeless plight) slept in the Mess tent, & the next morning orders came for us to move into our present huts. They are funny little boxes 6×16 ft., the most flimsy affairs, made of single canvas with Mica windows. The sides open out, & in fact in cool weather they feel completely open. It is a relief having a floor under us. They look exactly like little Noah's Arks. Each sister has one to herself. Lollie & I have amalgamated ours – one is a bedroom & the other called a sitting room, though more of a general junk room.

We continue to be busy all the time, having to send out patients to the Convalescent Camp who are really unfit to go, but we have to have the beds for sicker people.

The new huts the patients are in are very nice. There are four "lines" – each line composed of three huts – each hut accommodating 45. Each Sister has a hut of her own, & it is quite a work, for there is all the ordering & executive work, which if the three huts were in one, could be done by one person. It seems as though each one of us does so much work that could have been avoided with a little forethought on the part of those designing the place. However in many ways it is awfully nice having one's own hut to arrange the work without assistance or interference.

All my patients are so nice. They all seem so happy – one rarely hears grumbling – they are so thankful to get into a bed & away from the strain that everything seems delightful for them. It is terrible how short we are of reading matter. I took down a lot of old Gazettes & Stars[48] – six weeks old – & the Men have been devouring them. It is pathetic to see these Australians, New Zealanders, & Englishmen reading Goodwin's advertisements!![49]

You may notice my notepaper is rather varied. I have run out of my stock, so fell back on some Red Cross paper we got for the patients, & then found this odd sheet. I feel mean using the Red Cross paper for it cuts short the Men. We have written to England for some, so hope soon to have a supply.

There are rumours about that we may not be here very long. Whether that is merely hearsay, I don't know. I feel we are doing good work & am glad to stay as long as we are needed. The report goes that the authorities have decided after having put ten hospitals on the Island that it is not fit for them & now no surgical cases are to be landed. It is a queer affair, & everyone feels more or less unsettled.

I feel that this is a very stupid letter, but one cannot say all that one would like to – for reasons.

Hoping you are all well & with Much love
        Affectionately yours.
            Mildred H. Forbes.

Letter No. 27
Lemnos
October 27th, 1915.

Dear Mother,

I can hardly believe it is a week ago yesterday since I wrote you last. [N]ow that the evenings are so cold, we go to bed almost directly we get off, in order to keep warm, & so there seems no time for letter writing....

...

In one sense our work is not awfully hard, except for the rather long hours, for we do little heavy work, the orderlies doing that for us, but the work *is worrying*; everyone is more or less up against it, there is a shortage on all sides, & one can only do the best they can with what they've got – & even that has to be fought for day in & day out – the hardest fighter

& worst kicker usually coming out on top. It is most wearing! Then the climate un-doubtably affects one, for there is no doubt the whole unit individually is irritable & high strung. Everyone seems ready to fly off the handle on the slightest provocation!!! And yet not one of us would go back if we could under present conditions. The hospital is always full, & a bed no sooner empty, then another patient is admitted. How they manage to be around "the corner" all the time is beyond me, for each camp is a great distance apart.

Our patients are all either dysentery, jaundice or typhoid. [T]he latter as soon as possible are transferred to one of the General Hospitals, where there are more nurses, & they are rather better equipped & so able to look after such patients to better advantage, so that means *our* place is filled with dysentery, & so day after day one goes through the same routine, giving the same medicines & treatments!! You can understand the monotony. If it wasn't for the constant change of patients, I don't know how we could stand it, especially as the improvement is so slow. I can't understand *why* the climate should be so un-healthy, unless the sudden change in temperature is the cause of it; of course at first the sanitary precautions for the troops were not – well perhaps it is as well not to enlarge. But it's a sandy soil, there are constant winds & that always means trouble.

Our hospital seems to have come to a stand-still as regards being enlarged, & a General Hospital about ½ mile from us being pushed forward. The latter's huts are a great improve[ment] on ours – windows more numerous, made to open decently with a kind of arrangement to avoid draughts – places at the end of each hut for two baths & two lavatories, whereas our poor men have quite a walk to the latrine, that is those who are able to get out of bed. When one sees these immense places being built, one can't help but doubt the rumours one hears regarding the withdrawing of men from the Dardanelles.

Surely no one will ever bother reading this far.[50] I wish I could tell you more, but it is wiser not to go into too much detail. I am most anxious to hear how many of my letters have *really reached* you.

Yesterday we had the A.D.M.S. inspect the place, & everyone was made to put their best foot forward. I'd love to tell you what I really think of his criticisms. Imagine on *active service*, where everyone has more work than they can do, & the men owing to this doing much for themselves when they are too sick to care what happens, having the cleanliness of their feet criticised!!! Orderlies ordered to keep their beds in a straighter line!!!

It makes me sick. Of course no-body pays any attention, but goes bliss-fully on doing the best they can, but when you stop to think it does make one mad. I believe it is his first time on Active Service & he would like to see the place kept like the Military Hospitals in times of peace, when they have an orderly to every patient practically, whereas we have two for 45 patients, & often only one.

Oh! I wish I could talk to you instead of writing, for one can only touch on everything, & then probably have given altogether a different impression to what one intended.

...

By the way at last the Red Cross are sending us a few odds & ends, the English branch of course.... I am sure we don't get half that we should, but don't know whether it is our Officers' fault who go after it or whether [the Red Cross] favor their own hospitals more. Am inclined to think the latter. The Australians of course have their Red Cross headquarters at Cairo, so they are well looked after.

...

Always love dear to you, from Yours lovingly
Lollie.

[P.S.] ...

Letter No. 28
Lemnos
October 30th, 1915

Dear Mother,

...

A Stationary Hospital is entitled to 26 Sisters & a Matron, but is only supposed to accommodate 250 to 300 patients, while we have always 600, & sick ones at that.[51] Of course we can't evacuate quite so often here as in France, as patients can only leave in great numbers when a hospital ship comes in port – then if the weather is bad, & the winds high, it is impossible in these troublesome waters to load or un-load. Even supply ships are sometimes kept days in the harbour, owing to its being impossible to have them un-loaded. Of course it all has to be done by "lighters,"[52] as there are no wharves or docks worth speaking of, & the breezes here often do damage to those we have.

I'm so anxious to get a reply to my Lemnos letters, & am rather wondering what impressions you get from what I said. There is much that is beautiful, more that is interesting but un-mentionable, but in spite of all this, I don't think one could paint conditions blacker than they actually were, &

I might almost add are, for while the improvements, especially as regards ourselves, are many, the general management of affairs is beyond understanding.... As you will know by now we came to nothing but contaminated ground & a well full of germs – but brought all our equipment with us – a very badly chosen one at that....

...

... The past few days have been quite warm again, the sort of heat one dislikes, rather sticky & depressing, although the sun has not been so intense, consequently have not minded it particularly. It always means unfortunately a set-back for our dysentery cases, & after such weather, new patients admitted usually have a worse form of the trouble than those admitted during a cool spell. This weather also means an increase in flies, much to our regret!

By the way there has been a good deal of trouble regarding what has been written home about conditions here, & while I'm rather glad, in fact *more* than glad, that things are being talked about from the house tops, it means that in future the *Canadian* letters will in all probability be rather strictly censored. Am wondering if even this will reach you. Just why we shouldn't mention personal discomforts & lack of supplies for patients is beyond me, & think it shows someone must have a very un-easy conscience in objecting to it.

Of course the point is that the Canadian Red Cross have been most liberal if all accounts are true in France, but out here we are strictly under British Red Cross & so far the supply has been very inadequate, & it evidently is being looked into. The whole affair is too intricate for me, but no doubt owing to all the red tape attached to every new move, & the fact that none of our own men are here, our Canadian Red Cross are not represented out here. All I know is that we haven't got what we should have. Time will tell why. It certainly isn't owing to the lack of generosity of the public, for there are plenty of supplies & comforts of all kinds at headquarters, & as fast as they are used are re-newed – the trouble has been in the distribution. There are other points but [the] less said the better.

...

Yours lovingly
Lollie.

P.S. Mildred says to be sure & give you her love. She is now indulging in her *weekly* sponge.

Lemnos
Letter No. 29
November 4th, 1915

Dear Mother,

...

   We have been having great lectures on not saying too much in our
letters, so if they sound a little restrained at times & rather lack news, you
will understand why. If they only thought a minute, they would realize
now there was not any necessity to grumble as at first, for conditions
are so much better, especially from a personal standpoint, but from the
patients', there is a great need for improvement as far as food is concerned.
We are always running short of various things, owing I suppose to supplies
not arriving on the island, & there is never anything else to replace the
lacking article.

   I know in my small Ward of 45 patients, they hadn't had an egg for three
days, & [I] managed to get some by sending an orderly over to the village.
It meant I spent 10 shillings & each patient had *one* egg. Of course I can't
afford to keep it up in the first place, & in the second, if we all did it,
there aren't enough eggs on the island to supply us.... [I]t is only a question
of days I suppose before more arrive, but in the meantime, it means just
bread & jam for tea for the patients who are allowed that – but the majority being dysentery get just a little arrow-root & cup of tea. Of course it
doesn't *sound* bad, but as the diet *never* varies you can imagine how sick
they get of it.

Nov. 6th

...

   To-night we have quite a satisfied feeling for once again the laundry
man has been, & we have got rid of our dirty linen. It's the hardest work to
get any laundry done, & when it comes back it's difficult sometimes to tell
whether they have touched it. Nothing is ironed so you can imagine how
quickly everything gets soiled again.

...

   Yours lovingly
   Lollie

Lemnos
November 6th, 1915

My dear Cairine,

Your last letter received was from St. Andrews, where you seemed to be enjoying it very much. I tried to picture you all there. Am so glad the summer was a happy one....

We are having the most beautiful days – lovely clear skies, and just enough coolness in the air to make it pleasant. It reminds me of May or early September at home. The nights are very cold, & yet a *heavy* dew falls. The changes are extraordinary here....

With the cooler weather & better food, etc. we are all (the nursing sisters) much better & happier. Things have improved considerably though still we hope for better conditions.

Up to this we have been very busy, but for the last couple of days I personally have had a very easy time. We have sent a lot of patients to the Base, others to Convalescent Camp, & we have not had many admissions, due, I expect to the good weather. A bad storm will mean intense suffering at the Peninsula, & consequently we get a lot of sick men.

No surgery is coming to this Island, so we don't get heavy work. Dysentery is the chief disease, so it means a good deal of routine work. I go about with a large bottle (once used for Whiskey) now filled with a mixture which ¾ of my patients get. The shortage at times of food for the Men is terrible. They have not had eggs for at least five days, & porridge also has not been obtainable. It means for the men who are comparatively well, bread, (always more or less sour) & jam. I hate to see meals being served. Eggs of sorts can be bought in the neighboring villages – five for one shilling – usually three out of the five will be bad. Some of the sisters have been buying eggs themselves for the Men, but ... the price mentioned to provide for 45 Men makes it rather high, for one egg is not going to cure or "feed up" a patient & one cannot afford to provide them continually. Anyway I don't approve of the plan at all. I believe three supply ships were sent to this Island, but got to the wrong one!

Well, the "public holiday" November 18th will soon be here.[53] We expect to have a round of gaiety, as Cecily Galt's birthday is on the 10th, Lollie's the 14th. We three wrote a long time ago home saying we expected food for the festivities – so far nothing has arrived, & I fear it won't, as parcels take ages to drift in here. However we three among ourselves will strive to celebrate!

Lollie & I had a great trip on donkeys the other day. We had a "day off" from 10:00 so decided to try & get away from the Camp, which I, for one, am rather sick of. We took one of the orderlies with us for protection, & started off mounted on ... donkeys, with a small Greek aged about 15 running after us. As a matter of fact he did not have to *run* much, for the donkey's pace was not alarming!

We took a mountain trail to a tiny place called Therma. The trip itself was splendid – the country in spite of all its barrenness, is very attractive, though *not* beautiful (except when the sun sets & then it is simply glorious). We got to the village – if one can call it one. There are about three straggling houses, one of which is a "hotel." The Rockland ones are Ritz Carltons[54] in comparison. Lunch ... was a frightful meal. (We ate it outside with the farm-yard inhabitants assisting us to do away with the food – they got most of it).... But I wanted to tell you [that] before our collation we had a *bath* – something quite unusual here!

There are sulphur springs in Therma, the water being almost boiling. In this queer ... hotel they have a bath room fixed up. All very primitive. There is a marble floor, & the hot sulphur water comes out of a pipe, a piece of wood being used for a plug. Here one takes pans full of water to splash about to get accustomed to the heat before descending to the bath. It is sunk below the level of the floor, also made of marble. Sounds grand, but I assure you it isn't! However I got a lovely hot bath & soaked for ages, feeling luxurious. One felt though things looked terrible, that with that hot water constantly flowing over the marble, it ought to be fairly clean.

If we could get an eatable meal there, it would be splendid to go for the sake of the tub.

Well, I must close for now. With Much love to all

Affectionately yrs. Mildred H. Forbes

Letter No. 30
Lemnos
November 14th, 1915[55]

Dear Mother,

... [Y]esterday we had another mail, a fine big one, bringing my birthday letter from you dated Oct. 12th.... [I]t has made such a difference in my birthday.... Of course I'm just dying to get the parcels, but am afraid it may be some time yet before they arrive, for every available boat ... is being used for other purposes, & transport is most difficult from every point....

The eats sounds great, & while conditions have improved tremendously, & food in particular, biscuits are 2/s [per pound],[56] poor ones at that & only attainable at times – in fact the same can be said of almost everything except government rations, & even those we don't get in full. However we have *plenty* of a sort, but the extras will be more than acceptable, & my tongue is literally hanging out for a piece of Mr. Claxton's birthday cake! We simply had to tell one another about the prospective parcels!

Homemade candy sounds luscious & tooth paste will be more than acceptable. I'm just dying to get it.... It is such a joy getting things I am tempted to accept your offer of a small weekly package. You've no idea how acceptable & exciting every small package is!! And I can't think of anything that isn't acceptable.

...

... Galt's ... birthday ... on the 10th was a decided failure. Firstly she was sick in bed with a bilious headache, secondly, no mail arrived & no pack-ages. So Mildred & I after scouring the country came back with only some ginger snaps! These were presented in style! To-day, my birthday is a decided improvement. I have had mail, & while no eatables or parcel have arrived, we have arranged an impromptu supper for 9 p.m. for three of us.

Cocktails. (½ whiskey ½ water)
Hors d'oeuvre (potted meat on unsweetened biscuits, Lipton's & punk!)
Lobster with biscuits. (The same biscuits! A small tin of lobster we found in a canteen.)
Champagne Jelly. Our sweet! made in the Ward from flat Champagne left in a bottle from a patient who couldn't drink the same. (This was a failure. Didn't set!!!)
Walnuts, milk chocolate (by way of dessert).
Liqueur (Brandy stolen from the Wards).
Canadian Cigarettes presented to me by Mildred before leaving home.

This is a great event & has required a great deal of thought to prepare. Mildred, as you know, celebrates on the 18th & we live in hopes of at least one parcel arriving before then.

...

Judging by the papers, the men in this part of the world have everyone's sympathy now. As a man writing to the "Times" says, they are up against it in every way, & the un-fortunate part is few of these difficulties can be over-come such a distance from home.

...

The other day the island had a visit from "my friend" [Kitchener] whose photo I sent.... This visit ought to have some good results, ones we can already feel. I didn't see him, as his interest is not specially in hospitals.[57]

...

... [T]he work here is so different from France – no large convoys arriving & then a slackening up, but ... a steady flow coming in to the hospital just as fast as the beds are vacated. The work, now that things have more or less righted themselves, is not fearfully hard, just steady, but it is rather depressing & one feels un-satisfactory. I do wish we could get better *food* for the patients.

By the way there have been all kinds of troubles regarding the censoring of letters – I do hope I haven't said too much for this to be sent on. Certainly I have given no information of use to the enemy, although the Censor may think I am criticising, which is I am told an offence from a military standpoint!!! Just why we shouldn't write for the things the patients need I fail to see. Can't tell you all the trouble there has been – that will have to keep until I get home.

One thing I can't understand is the Censor having the patience to read my epistles! Hence I occasionally take chances – not that I have mentioned the many interesting things that I would like to.

...

Mildred is quite herself again, but still a regular target for fleas; not being in any too good a condition & an ardent scratcher, she has many wounds, several of which have got infected in turn!!! In any other country one might be worried, but here we realize the cause. It is only too common.

Well good-night. I do hope you are getting my letters fairly regularly.... Heaps of love always & in case of delays a very happy Xmas, although I do hope to write a Christmas letter later.

...

Lollie.

Letter No. 31
Lemnos
November 19th, 1915

Dear Mother,

Just four days ago I sent you off an un-usually lengthy epistle, enclosing a cheque for your Xmas present, but knowing how un-certain all mail is,

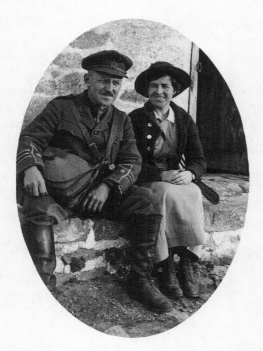

Colonel Williams and Nursing Sister Mildred Forbes at the shrine
on Mount Therma, taken by Nursing Sister Laura Holland. *UBC
Archives, Laura Holland fonds*

particularly lately, thought I would write again sooner than usually, hoping
one or the other will reach you in time to wish you a very happy Xmas, if
perhaps rather a lonely one, & that 1916 will prove a much happier one for
everyone & you in particular.

...

On the 16th Mildred & I were given our day off for this week, & were
starting off at 11 a.m. with our lunch under our arms for a place about
3 miles off ... when we were over-taken by our O.C., Major Williams, who
asked to join us.... [W]e waited while he got & added his share to our
luncheon parcel, decided as we had a cavalier to change our course & go
on what is more or less forbidden ground when alone ... the highest point
on the island ... [W]hile it was a long walk ... (7 miles each way) up-hill &
a pretty rough climb at the end, we were more than rewarded by the sight
which greeted us on our arrival. Here, as on the top of all the hills on the

island, was the usual Shrine – very tumble-down & primitive in appearance
– & the view showing the *whole* of the island, with the entire shore, most
of the valleys, & various surrounding smaller islands. Being a beautifully
clear day, we could see in the distance quite distinctly the cliffs on the Asia
Minor coast & also the outline of some of the Grecian islands. Major
Williams has a splendid camera & took several snaps. He has promised
me some prints as soon as he can find time to develop them, so will send
them as soon as possible.

...

Yours lovingly
Lollie.

[P.S.] ...

Letter No. 32
Lemnos
November 23rd, 1915

Dear Mother,

There is a chance of my being able to get this posted in London through
a semi-friend, thus avoiding any censorship, & so feel free-er to discuss
various things otherwise impossible. Just at present we have ... to be particularly careful, as a good deal of trouble has been caused by an in-discreet
parent taking up the cause of "his child", regarding conditions on our
arrival.[58] Being a "man of affairs" he was listened to – the government took
it up – inquiries cabled to England, then here, & the whole affair has been
looked into by the G.O.C., the A.D.M.S., D.D.M.S. & the D.M.S. etc.,
etc. Of course all this fuss has made each one mad in turn, & yet nothing
was written that was not perfectly true, & in no way was anything mentioned "of interest to the enemy." We all, Officers as well as Sisters, wrote
home much the same news, but in most cases it has gone no further. Of
course there is no doubt about it, the mis-management of affairs has been
colossal, & in consequence everyone has & is suffering for it. It's all very well
to say it is what one must expect on active service – & we are all willing to
put up with hardships that can't be avoided – but when it can be remedied
why suffer in silence? ... [I]t doesn't do to go into details but I feel confident
the next colonial hospital unit sent out from England to new fields won't
start out in quite the ignorance of what is necessary as the first to come here.

Men keep coming & going from here, the population of our *own kind* varying from 30,000 to 42,000, all camping within a small area. [Y]ou can imagine what a sight it is both by day & after dark when the camp fires are burning. This number does not include any of the many hospitals, their personnel or patients.

...

... Military life is certainly the devil – the whys & the wherefores are incomprehensible to any & everybody – & never supposed to be noticed; no one is expected to take any responsibility, but to shift it on to someone else. [C]onsequently often work is neglected because no one seems to be responsible for it, & rather than interfere with another's work, it is left un-done. However daily I am learning more & more to hold my tongue, & am afraid by the time I get back home, I shall practically have become dumb. [F]ortunately having Mildred, I can let off steam occasionally & so not altogether lose the art of making myself heard.

The other day we had an invite to an afternoon concert on board one of the battleships, so arranged to have afternoon hours off duty & went, & certainly it was a wonderful sight. The crew had got up a minstrel show, for which they had been practising for several months. A proper stage with electric foot lights ... had been built on the aft deck, which must have been cleared somewhat, for with the exception of two immense guns, it was quite empty of all obstacles, & enough chairs arranged for several hundred sailors. They are, especially when seen in numbers, a fascinating looking lot of men, much more so really than the Tommies. After the concert the Officers served tea, & altogether it was very nice. We really get a number of invites one way & another on board the boats, but it takes such a time to get there & back that usually one can't conscientiously spare the time.

The hospital at present is full, but not so heavy as it has been – however we were informed just two days [ago] to be prepared to take in any number, that a rush was expected & in case of necessity we might have to empty store-huts, double up the personnel & so make extra room. [H]owever there is no use worrying ahead, in fact am becoming quite placid, or I might say "Military" in my attitude, that what must be, must be; if you have no com-forts to give a man, he must do without.... It's sickening but the attitude of many un-fortunately, though of course there are hundreds who think, feel & act differently.

Every few days we see several hundred men starting off after a few weeks rest on the island, back again to the front – headed at times by a band – their equipment on their back, their uniform, anything but uniform in their dilapidated condition. It just brings a lump in your throat – this endless snake-like line of men, & yet we know how few will return. [I]t is appalling how many men tell you that originally they belonged to a regiment of from 1,000 to 1,200 men, of which perhaps only a hundred or so remain.

We have been having a number of miserably cold days lately – just like November at home, only accompanied by tremendously high & persistent winds. Of course living practically out of doors as we are at present makes us realize a change in the weather much more than at home. Last night in spite of sitting with our heavy blue sweaters & policeman's coat[s] on, we were shivering, & finally filled two hot water bottles, got in our red dressing gowns & under the invaluable Jaeger blankets[59] before we could get warm. To-day each hut has been presented with a small coal oil stove, & it makes a tremendous difference, for at least we can get our hands warmed. It's very hard on the patients, for their wooden huts are badly built, & in no way heated, but of course this weather won't last, & on days when the sun shines & the air is still one can forget the nights.

Unfortunately the colder the night, the greater the necessity for me about 2 a.m. to visit the "Latrine." At this hour the conventional one is ignored, & in spite of a bright moon, we glance around to see that no guard is in sight, trust to luck & "perform" at our very door. These windy nights am afraid our clothes have suffered somewhat in consequence. Even suppose they could provide us with proper utensils, it would be simply impossible to empty them, for one can never even get to the "latrine" except in view of half a dozen men. I no longer feel self-conscious passing men in my dressing gown & stockingless legs, for this is my first walk in the morning, but have not yet the courage to carry a jerry of any description even if it were obtainable. To-day I did knock the narrow neck off a cheap earthen ware jug, & shall use it on *very* stormy nights.

...

Well dear, I am afraid you will think I am doing nothing but criticise – but who can I talk to this way if not to you?

Much as I long for the War to be over, & once again to be back enjoying the comforts of home (& some days we feel pretty desperate), still I really am wonderfully happy in the work, & feel it is much easier for us who are busy out here, than for those working at home. Mildred says to tell you she can really see me putting on *fat* – certainly I eat enough to keep two women alive. But in spite of it all I've never had the energy to wash my hair! You can imagine the state it is in!!!

... Heaps of love to you always & love to Uncle George from Lollie.

Letter No. 33
Lemnos
November 28th, 1915

Dear Mother,

...

Last night in this awful weather,[60] thirteen new Sisters arrived from London.... [O]nly two days ago there was an order (very much resented by us all) from higher authority than our own that the Sisters were to come off night duty; consequently this gives us several *extra* Sisters on day duty, & means that until the place is enlarged, extra help is not needed. Poor girls, my heart aches for them, coming out at such a time & to such weather before they have ... got into the run of things.... [T]oo many on the job ... only means we'll have to do orderly work. Of course when the place is enlarged they really will be needed, & if the expected rush comes, it will be a god-send.

In the meantime the situation is difficult to explain in a letter going through the hands of a Censor, especially of our own unit, for much of it would be mis-understood. I am afraid many of our Officers think the Sisters a bally nuisance, & I'm willing to admit that we are, for when we see a pos-sibility of small improvements, we kick & fuss until we get them – the kind of comforts that men who are *well* & strong don't think necessary, but a woman realizes they make *all* the difference, & un-doubtably shorten the convalescent period. I will never make an ardent advocate of equal rights for women, for if the War has taught me one thing it is that certain work can only be properly done by women, & other work by men. Of course the difficult point to decide, & over which the both sexes would have many arguments, is just which part *is* a woman's work, & which part a man's. In hospital work, a man only wants to leave to the women the menial work which he detest[s] doing himself, & if forced to do does it very badly, al-though he has wonderful ideas how *women* should do it!!

...

My love to Uncle George. I do hope he isn't going to make himself ill worrying over Temple. The way the war is lasting, it was inevitable he should come sometime, & I'm so glad he was able to volunteer when he did, for he certainly would have regretted it all his life if he had done otherwise. The remarks passed by the men now regarding the men who have stayed at home are not pleasant, & when the war is over & they are back home, feel sure the stay-at-homes will be shunned.

Well I *must* stop. Seem to be wound up to-night. Heaps & heaps of love dear to you always. Don't worry, & while I must admit at times I do feel lonely & long to see you, yet on the whole am very happy.

Lovingly Lollie.

Lemnos
December 5th, 1915

My dear Cairine,

...

... I am on night duty just now. Am putting in two weeks, & how I hate it. This is my third night of it. Luckily for me Lollie is on too. I get so fearfully sleepy, & the nights seem endless.

We had such a cold snap a week ago. I think it was forerunner of joys to come. First it blew a hurricane, then it rained & then froze so hard that the water froze solid in the fire bucket outside my hut.

We suffered terribly with the cold as the wind sifted right in to our huts. They supplied us with coal oil heaters – also gave us each a sweater, puttees and a heavy Khaki coat, the kind the cavalry people wear. I was so bundled up could hardly move. Well, we may have found it cold but our misery is nothing compared to what the poor Men suffered at the Front. They were in seven feet of water – those who were not drowned climbed on to a ledge in the trenches & there stood for 36 hours in three feet of water.

The result is we have any number of Men in with frozen feet. If they had only known enough to take off their puttees, a great deal of trouble could have been averted. They must have suffered with the cold most terribly & am afraid it is going to be even worse next month.

We are still eagerly looking out for the supplies which are being sent us. I hope they will get here before Xmas.

...

This is a short stupid letter, but am so sleepy & have no news.

With much love & best wishes for 1916 to you all. Affectionately yours Mildred H Forbes.

Letter No. 37.
Lemnos.
December 20th, 1915

Dear Mother,

...

You can have no conception of the general feeling of un-rest & the fearful depression that meets us on every side. Everyone is "fed up" to the greatest extent, & yet strange to say we would all be fearfully disappointed if moved before our troops leave this quarter of the globe.

I am tremendously interested in hearing what the outside world thinks of this wonderful retreat from the Peninsula. Just at present we here feel it will go down in history as one of the great events of the war, & yet it is *not* although so near, quite understandable, for it has been a tremendous surprise both to us here, & the men themselves who have come down from the trenches. Of course the possibility of an evacuation has been a rumour for ages, & towards the middle of last week, we realized, an authentic one.

Yesterday about 8 a.m. we noticed a large number of troops winding along the main road (a few yards back of our quarters), towards the Detail Camp, when it dawned on us they might be the men from the Peninsula, so four of us rushed for cigarettes we had in our huts for Xmas, & tore up to give them to these men. It was a wonderful sight – their delight at seeing anyone in the female line, their eagerness for the smoke. [S]uch weary, dust stained, white faced humanity; many told us they had been seventeen weeks in the trenches without ever coming out!!! In this country that means nothing but bully-beef, jam, & hard biscuits with occasionally soup & bread. One quart of water is their allowance for 24 hours for tea, soup, etc., many shaving themselves with the dregs of their tea – a wash is practically unknown – & yet they were wonderfully cheerful, their one regret being that they had had to leave what they had fought so hard to get.

I ran into the Australians from Anzac, two of the other girls into some of the English troops, & our 2,000 cigarettes seemed like giving a pound of candies to a thousand children.

Of course as you can well understand, everything in this country is apt to be a bit irregular, but even we were rather surprised that the men, on seeing us ready to distribute cigarettes, dropped out of line & clamoured around us. It wasn't long before the senior officer shouted for the men of A Company to fall into line, when Brock, one of our girls & quite a character, shouted, "Have A Company all cigarettes"!! Everyone nearly took a fit.

I'm not a scrap in a letter writing mood, much as I long to talk to you, & so feel I am giving you no idea of the scene, but it's well imprinted on my mind, & so you will have it all some day. The rear-guard are supposed to have got off alright last night, & of course long before you get this, the papers will have told how not a shot was fired. Here we had expected a tremendous influx of wounded, & not one [has] arrived. Of course now we all are wondering what next? Surely all these hospitals won't be needed now that there are so few men at the Peninsula.

...

Since coming off night duty I have been put in the Mess to help Upton, as the work especially around Xmas time is too much for one individual; I hate it & find I come off duty each night with my brain in a whirl & my nerves on edge. The endless talking, growling, & up-set is awful. We are however going to have a wonderful Xmas dinner, & through various kind naval friends have managed to get quite a lot of stuff – at any rate turkey, extra vegetables, etc. A large order given by one war-ship in harbour to a transport boat has fallen to our lot (of course we paid for it) as the said boat has since departed to other seas.... Will write regarding Xmas doings in a day or so, but want this to go to-night. Love to Uncle George. A whole heap for your own self

from Yours lovingly
Lollie.

[P.S.] ...

Letter No. 38
Lemnos
December 28th, 1915

Dear Mother,

I can hardly believe it is eight days since I wrote you last, but ... knowing how rushed we were around Xmas time, no doubt my memo book[61] is correct.... [O]nly *one* of the Sisters received parcels from England, in spite of each one of us having sent an order weeks ago for decorations, small presents, etc., & very few parcels of any kind arrived in time. The Red Cross sent a few odds & ends, a small package for each patient containing soap, a wash cloth, two boxes cigarettes, matches & a little writing paper, & there were a few Xmas puddings.... However through navy friends, the Mess Order from Malta arrived & we made the most of the little we had, the patients entered into the spirit of it all & really did wonders – the result was a surprise to everyone ...

... [T]he Sisters provided potatoes & squash ... for [the patients'] dinner, also nuts & oranges ... & the government provided roast beef.... The Sisters also managed to buy enough eggs for them both for breakfast & tea, besides a few little extras, one hut having butter for one meal, another biscuits – just what we could manage ... & really the men were more than grateful & realized we had done what we could on this miserable isle...

... [W]e wanted to remember the men of the unit in some small way, & so bought muslin in the village & made a small bag for each man, filling it with everything we could lay our hands on. Each man received candies, oranges, nuts, cigarettes, a pipe, a handkerchief & one other article, such as mouth organ, shaving soap, writing pad, etc.

Brock ... undertook to decorate the Men's Mess Tent & on Xmas Eve ... Colonel Williams called a special parade, gave them a Xmas address, & we handed out their bags, each one having [the man's] own name on it. As there were 139 men, it meant quite a lot of work ... in spite of each man receiving so little, but I know they appreciated our having done what we could.

...

We didn't attempt to do anything in our own Mess Tent on Xmas day.... [E]ach girl spent every minute in the hospital & scarcely took time to come up for her meals – in fact all my time seemed to be spent giving a bite to each one when-ever they could manage to come up. Also Upton & I did what we could towards getting things ready for the following day, when we had our own Xmas dinner. And really it was a wonderful success. We decorated the place with red paper that had been used by the Men's Mess the day previously [&] had a candle lantern hanging over each table with ribbon streamers coming down ... to each place....

Upton managed to get the turkeys on the island two weeks previous, & ... while they were rather skinny, tasted mighty good. All the other things really came from Malta, an order sent by one of the battleships for us, & through their energies arrived here on time. Really I don't know how we ever would have existed if it hadn't been for these naval men. Of course they have opportunities of getting supplies in a way that no one else has, & as they live well themselves, sympathize with we poor creatures on shore. Then of course we have several very pretty girls in our unit & that has helped more than a little.

Just here I may mention our Matron didn't get back from Cairo until to-day,[62] & none of us had any regrets, for we were able to manage our Christmas affairs just as we all wanted to do.

On the Monday, the hospital being very light since the exodus Christmas day, we gave a small tea, inviting the officers from surrounding Camps who at different times had sent us invitations to small teas etc. It was a great success, between 75 & 100 officers coming – there was plenty to eat & the tent looked very pretty, in the dim candle light. Naturally this meant lots of work for Upton & self.... [A]ll this sounds as though we were having a round of festivities, but [it] being so difficult to do anything makes a small affair seem to us quite magnificent!

...

... I hate to mention your boxes for I know just how disappointed you will be to hear they've never arrived, but I don't at all give up hope regarding them, & much as I would love to have had the things for Xmas, feel that a little later on they will be even more acceptable.

...

This letter will have to be censored so can't tell you all the interesting tales I have heard the past few days about the evacuation. I wonder just what the papers will say about it.

When writing before we weren't quite sure what to believe, but since then we have had facts from beginning to end, told by men there on the spot from start to finish & in a position to really see what was doing.... [C]ertainly the whole thing was wonderful, not only as regards well laid plans, but apparent ignorance on the enemy's side, splendid weather conditions, etc.

...

I'm afraid you're doing altogether too much – now do look after yourself, for with a daughter of 32 you can't be as young as you used to be!

Always love to you. I've missed you terribly this Xmas season but cheered myself with the thought that we'll be together next year.

Mildred sends love also. Yours lovingly
   Lollie.

Lemnos
December 31st, 1915

My dear Cairine,

It is hard to realize that this is the last day of 1915. One wonders what the next year will be like. Today is so warm it seems like a day in early September. We hear of the bad weather but it has kept off remarkably well – no doubt when it does come we will not be spared much.

... None of us have seen the artesian wells you speak of – however there is a large condensor by the Harbour, so we get a fair supply of water. Even then all drinking water *must* be boiled – one rarely has a drink of water, for by the time it is boiled, it is rather precious as well as having a queer taste. I wish we could import some of your good Rockland water!

In spite of all the boxes shipped us over two months ago, none of them have arrived. It takes ages for large boxes to reach us.

We are all feeling rather unsettled, for last week we thought we might have a move, but now it does not seem as though things were going that way. It is a fearful disappointment, for one's hopes were raised. Not that I really object to this place, but a change is always welcome, & four months of Lemnos is quite enough. I dread the thought of another hot season here. Oh, well, lots may happen before then.

Christmas passed off very successfully, especially from the patient's standpoint. With the usual luck of a Hospital, it proved to be a very busy day. One of the large Hospital ships was in, & decided to load up on Xmas. Our patients (a number from my ward included) were ready for the ambulances at 7 a.m. & did not go off till 6 p.m!! So you can imagine it was a long trying day for them – but their delight at getting "home" was pathetic. Most of the poor creatures had terrible feet due to frost bites – some had had their feet amputated here – the others will be sure to lose theirs.

...

There was plum pudding supplied by Lady Hamilton's Gift Fund, & we all bought vegetables for the patients, for the poor souls never get a vegetable here. So they had potatoes, squash, & beets. Potatoes are $8.00 a bag here! so they are rather a luxury! We have them for our Mess, but we are now living quite comfortably....

All the wards were decorated & looked remarkably well. I hadn't a thing to put up, & no ideas. However the day before Xmas managed to secure some red triangular handkerchiefs, which we knotted together & draped around the hut, then took absorbent cotton & made "Merry Xmas" etc. & stuck the letters on with vaseline. We got hold of some queer looking cactus branches which the Men made into wreaths, which were hung in our windows. Altogether it was an attempt & it did not look badly.

We had our own Xmas dinner on Sunday night the 26th.

By the time this reaches you it will be around your birthday time. I will wish you many happy returns of February 4th & hope next celebration that I may be nearer you all.

Very Much love to all
 Affect. Yours. Mildred H. Forbes.

Letter No. 39
Lemnos
January 7th, 1916

Dear Mother,

It is simply impossible to describe Mildred's & my excitement when we
found ... that the long looked for packing cases had actually arrived. Captain
Johnston ... was already pulling out the first nails, so we rushed madly down
to look after our own, persuaded two good-natured officers to carry the seven
cases to our own hut, & then proceeded to peek at all in turn. We debated
whether we would un-pack or not, as we expect any day a hurry call to move
on, & I must say I was rather tempted to leave things as they were until we
reached our new hospital, the general feeling being that we will in all probability be dumped down in another such god-forsaken hole as we are in at
present. However Mildred's curiosity was too great, & I was only too eager
myself, & events have proved her right, for on coming to our wards this
morning ... found a great many patients who have had absolutely no extras
for Christmas.... [A]s several in all probability will go back to the fighting
line somewhere in a very short space of time, it has been lovely to give them
a few good eats, & to-morrow as far as possible will give them a Xmas bag
each, & so fill up the vacancies in their kit bag.

We lighted on my special box first – it arrived in perfect condition &
really I can't tell you how delighted I am – everyone has been kindness itself,
& when I think of all the time & thought you must have spent, for you
un-doubtably had the brunt of it all, I can't begin to thank you. Of course I
must confess I was fearfully disappointed nothing arrived on time for Xmas,
& even more so when I saw all the lovely things in the parcels. [A]nd yet
when I saw the delight of the patients to-day, for they felt they had not been
forgotten, [I] was indeed reminded it's "an ill wind" ... & really think they
appreciated everything almost more than if they had got them on Xmas
day itself.

At present the hospital is very light, only 16 in my hut instead of 40, so
am able to give them quite a good time. All the canned goods & hospital
supplies we are packing right up again, for no matter where we land, there is
always a tremendous shortage at first, difficulty in drawing from ordnance,
etc., & so we feel these things will help us out of many difficulties. I can't
thank everyone individually at once, but of course will do in time. Meanwhile try & thank everyone you can for us.... Such a windfall as it is – we've
seen nothing like it before, & everything we take out we pounce on as being
just what we wanted. Of course we haven't begun to take in what we really

have got, & won't until we un-pack again, but wanted you to know they had arrived!!!!

Of course I have forgotten what we were to expect, but have received ... seven cases between us. Am afraid my birthday one must have been lost as Captain Johnston says none of that lot have turned up at all.

Tell Uncle George the lamp is perfect & makes our evenings seem just twice as long, for our old lantern gave such a poor light, after one hour's reading or writing, I always had to give up. It works like a charm. It was one of the first things I came across, & having some oil in my hut immediately started it going.... You certainly are a star packer....

...

By the way I almost wept when I saw the teaspoons, they seemed so much like home – & was tickled to death about the glasses. One of the first things we both thought of in un-packing was the bottle of cocktail, & wouldn't go to dinner until we found it. Certainly Uncle surpassed himself when he mixed it; for once reality was even better than anticipation. I felt mine a little, but wonderful to relate (for the reverse is the rule), Mildred felt hers even more, & vowed she was in no condition to go to dinner! However she didn't disgrace the family or else I was too happy to notice it! To-night we celebrated *after* dinner by opening the cherry whiskey, & it is a drink truly fit for the Gods – Lemnos seems so much more attractive since.

Am afraid the box containing Mildred's "special" things from her sister has not arrived, but no doubt it will greet us at our destination – but she got five boxes of "comforts" for patients.... The khaki bags were splendid & meant so much to the receivers, although many of them are rather a poor class North country man or Scotchman, & so un-able from sheer reserve & shyness to express their thanks, & would find it even more difficult to write. If anyone feels disappointed that things are not acknowledged by the men themselves, do try & make them understand why. Mildred suggested it might be wise to put a small paragraph in the paper acknowledging the receipt of said boxes – but leave it entirely to your own discretion.

...

I know you must find it very provoking that we have never mentioned special articles needed – but for so long *everything* was needed, that it was difficult to enumerate the most important, & now our movements are so uncertain that again I hesitate, but should you get a cable saying we had arrived in some awful hole, a repetition couldn't be beaten (I don't mean of everything but *any* of the many things), with the exception of Malted Tablets & Oxo, both of which we can *now* get from ordnance.

...

Well I really must say good-night & good-bye for the present. Heaps of love dear & *many many* thanks, don't think I don't realize the endless hours you must have spent planning, asking and interesting people, packing, etc., to say nothing of all the lovely extras you yourself enclosed. The olives were a particularly thoughtful gift on your part, & already many have been devoured.

Hope soon to get another letter from you, also to be able to give you some definite news in my next.

Always yours lovingly
Lollie.

Letter. No. 40
Lemnos
January 15th, 1916

Dear Mother,

Thank goodness I am one of those fortunate beings not on duty – for it has poured with rain all night, I have been forced to move my bed three times in order to avoid the drips, & altogether feel I have spent a very restless & sleepless night, & am so thankful I can remain in my little canvas hut.... It is still coming down in torrents, & we have been forced to huddle our bits of furniture as much as possible into the middle of our room.... [I]f we are careful & keep our blankets & pillows from slipping on to the floor, by remaining in bed ... will be able to spend our day there more comfortably than anywhere. Oh! the comfort of having Washington Coffee[63] – biscuits & a few etc.'s in our room!

...

[Friday] turned out to be a gorgeous [day] – still cold for even walking we needed our sweaters & British Warms on, but it was bright & sunny, without a breath of wind. Hearing there was a fête on in Portianos, the village nearest to us, we wandered over to find the square a mass of British Tommies, & scarcely enough room for any of the natives. In all these small villages there is a small square, around which shops are put up, & beyond that houses scattered here & there. Always there is to be found an odd tree or so & a well. I imagine the latter usually accounts for the collecting to-gether of the houses near it.

After a time a space was cleared with the assistance of one of the British Mounted Police, who is always hovering around to keep an eye on the behaviour I imagine of the troops, & then a number of the Greeks danced a national dance of some description, some of them in the sheep skin coat & peculiar bloomer-pants typical of the natives, others in European clothes, & two of the Greek sailors.... The one musician kept good time although he brought forth no music on a queer little instrument which they call a lyre, but looks like a miniature cross between a violin & guitar with three strings. A number of the Greek girls usually perform ... but the immense crowd was too much for them, an interpreter apologising & saying they were too shy & bashful!

On the way home we hunted up the woman who has been doing our washing, as she had neglected sending home half the things we sent, & were greeted most courteously & invited up-stairs, where we found a spread on the table consisting of plates of nuts, ... raisins, & ... pasties.... We were offered small liqueur glasses with what appeared to be ... water, but we found strongly flavored with paregoric. Naturally we drank it all, but found when some Greeks came in they only take a sip & pass it on, the next visitor drinking out of the same glass. The Greeks tried to entertain us, then talked amongst themselves – we did like-wise & after fifteen minutes or so departed. Their only remarks in English were "English – good" "Canada *very good*," "Turk *no* good."

There is no furniture in their bedrooms at all, the bed clothing & mattress just being put on the floor, & during the day, if fine hangs out of the window, if not I imagine is folded neatly inside.... The actual home seems cleanly, the floors scrupulously clean, & there is no more furniture than is absolutely necessary. Apparently those who stay in all day wear shoes around the house, but if their foot gear is at all dusty or dirty, they retain the Eastern habit of leaving their shoes at the threshold, keeping on ... their stockings if they have any. Many of the men I notice don't wear stockings, using leggings & ... home-made shoes, resembling moccasins, made of some thin hide.

...

Heaps of love always from
       Lollie.

[P.S.] ...

Lemnos
January 21st, 1916

My dear Cairine,

A most lovely box arrived yesterday from London with your name enclosed. Everything in it is splendid. Amongst the articles is a most delicious cake, the best I have tasted for many a long day, then there is a tin of Galantine of Turkey,[64] which I know will be particularly good. I opened a tin of very good oxtail soup this morning & we had it for refreshment. It was a splendid box, and I cannot thank you enough for it.

I also received a letter from you yesterday dated November 24th – of course I have previously received one of a later date – but that is the way things go here. We can never tell when the mail is going to reach us.

We are half packed & just awaiting orders, but it may be a long time before we actually leave. It is boring work waiting about, & the sooner we go the better pleased I shall be. Yesterday we all moved out of our canvas huts & are now living en masse in some of the patients' vacated huts. It is not a change for the better, for although we are not very cramped, the noise is terrific, & one cannot get one moment's quietness.

We are having nice bright days. Slightly cold but the nights are fearfully cold. I go to bed with a rug & heavy Military coat over my Jaeger blankets doubled, & we are probably going to a hot climate, so it will be quite a change.

...

I think your Red Cross people have done wonders, but quite realize the amount of work you must do, getting them going, etc.

...

Well, I have no ideas – this life of enforced idleness is *very enervating*. With much love to you all, & ever so many thanks for the lovely box.

> Affectionately yours.
> Mildred H. Forbes

I never mentioned the $100.⁰⁰ your Circle have given for our Men here. It will be getting the things – anything will be welcome – for we are always ready to receive things, & can make such good use of them.

> Letter No. 41.
> Lemnos
> January 22nd, 1916

Dear Mother,

...

... We have only a handful of patients left, & expect most of them to leave to-day. That will only leave us a few Turkish prisoners, who we don't look after, except as regards doing their dressings. Such a decent-looking rather fine type of men, & certainly they are well looked after, & seem to be as happy as clams. It is remarkable what an impression they have made on the English Tommie – there seems to be no hard feeling at all, in fact quite the reverse, & all our men agree the Turks have been mighty decent enemies. Many are the tales told of give & take. At the evacuation of Helles, where in spite of the report to the contrary, the loss was between 400 to 700 men, an Officer told us how a few nights previous to leaving, they were trying to bury some of their dead, a Turk saw him & another man trying to reach an Officer, & being bright moonlight, they could see distinctly. The Turk deliberately put his rifle on the ground in front of him, showing he would not shoot, & so gave them their chance. This is only one of many similar tales. I was talking to one of the Navy men who was on the ship that was the last to leave after the evacuation of Suvla, & it was thrilling to hear him tell the story from beginning to end. Of course they all, as you know, got away most comfortably – no one seems to quite understand why – but it was quite different from what they anticipated.... [H]e said the tension on that ship was something awful, for had the enemy realized what was doing, & turned their big guns on them, they wouldn't have had any chance at all – not one had expected to get back alive. Well, it's all an old story now & I mustn't try to tell everything I know & hear on paper, or I'll have nothing to say when I get back.

... It is now January 24 – & we are still here. I am on duty in the Mess (where at present there is little to do) only every other day. In spite of having the whole day to ourselves, we seem to have no time for anything – being in a hut with 15 other girls means that we waste an immense amount of time, & when we attempt to either write or read are continually interrupted....
...

... [I]n regard to letters, while I feel it has been a great help to have my letters type-written & sent the rounds, ... I really think perhaps it would be wiser not to do so unless the receivers thoroughly understand, no matter of how little interest, it must not go any further.

It seems we are not allowed really according to military rules & regulations to discuss even the condition of our own hospital – everything except the scenery & sometimes even that is tabooed – needless to say no-body sticks to the restrictions, but un-fortunately some of the letters of this unit from both officers & sisters have got into the paper, the subject has been referred to England & a fuss made, giving our O.C. a lot of bother about nothing. Consequently we have had special warnings regarding these restrictions & are asked, particularly going to a new place, to be very careful that our home letters go no further than to our home people. Hence we are all sending these long rambling warnings.

The Western families I think have been the most indiscreet ones – no doubt in a small place the news-paper people on their own initiative, pick up scraps & put it in as a letter – anyways it's done. Lieutenant Colonel Elder does the same thing without an up-roar being made, it seems. Of course we're all sick of the subject here & no doubt you are too, so we'll say no more about it. Now that you understand the situation just do what you think best.

Every day we are not on duty we have breakfast in bed – most of the others do likewise, bringing bread & butter when there is any from dinner the previous night, all of us possessing either tea or coffee & a tin of milk of our own. This keeps us alive until lunch time, for which it is always difficult to be on time. In the afternoon we usually manage a good long walk, or if the weather is bad, read & try to get a few letters written, but the latter I find most difficult these days. There is absolutely nothing new, no chance of posting letters from now on until we reach Alexandria or some other port, & so one puts off letters from day to day.

The *latest* rumour says we go to *England!* I hope not but there's no use getting fussed for we won't know definitely until we have actually arrived. I hate the thought of the heat in Egypt, but like the work out here so much better. In England there is too much palavering to titled & influential people.

...

It has suddenly occurred to me that I have never told you about being moved out of our canvas huts into the empty wooden hospital huts, in order to get the former packed, as they go with us. In our hut there are 16 of us & in the other 22; just why we weren't divided equally is one of those mysteries our Matron continually gives us to solve....

...

The thought of all you are doing rather appalls me, & yet should we remain at this end of affairs, there is nowhere your efforts would be more appreciated. The only way to look at it is, one must always take more or less of a chance, & should we return to England, we will at any rate see that the *right* people get the things & our one regret will be that you spent extra money on freight.

Here we were routed out by one of the girls who wanted to get up a small party to go & have tea at the Egyptian Labor Camp, so as I was rather anxious to see the "gypies" at close quarters, Forbes & I went along. A number of Egyptians have been employed by the government to do laboring

work on the island, all of them of course volunteers & under military rules
& regulations as the carpenters are, but they are not soldiers. They have
done various kinds of work, such as the making of roads, breaking up of
stones, emptying latrines, etc. At one time they had between 6,000 & 7,000
of them here, [but] these have now dwindled down to about 1,300.

Their pay is 2/8 a day & of course the government provides them with
clothing, rations & sees that they are housed.... A camp of that type is rather
interesting to see; on account of their religion they bake their own bread
(really the same as ours, only made by their own cooks), import their animals
from Egypt for fresh meat (similar to lambs but ... different, I forget what
they call them), have beans one day, lentils the next, & rice by way of variety.
Never have they had such feeds in their life time before; on the other hand,
no doubt they have never worked so regularly or kept at it so steadily.

At first they lived in tents, now all are in small stone huts, packed away
on shelves like sardines, but it helps to keep them warm. They are filthy
dirty people ... & yet there is something so simple & childlike about them
one can't judge them the same as other people. They sing to & fro from work,
often when at it, grin & rush forward with delight whenever they see a
kodak,[65] & shirk work at every opportunity.

Having looked over the camp, had tea in the Officers' mess, a fearful
barracks of a place – but a mighty decent tea & nice enough men. The O.C.,
who I happened to be next, [is] an Englishman but has apparently spent the
largest part of his life in Egypt & loves the East. But of course at a tea of
that kind there is little chance of talking much, & I'm no hand at it anyway.
However enjoyed the affair on the whole....

January 26th, afternoon.

Yesterday I was on duty all day in the Mess so although there was not much
work to do could not leave the camp – especially as our cook had had rather
more than was good for him which made him quite forgetful, [so] had to
keep my eye on things in general. To-day was so lovely we decided to try &
catch the 11 a.m. ferry & go over to East Mudros, about the only place we
have not seen.... It is at East Mudros that the French troops & hospitals have
been stationed. Many have left during the past few weeks, but there are a
few camps left & one hospital, the latter a most un-attractive muddle of a
place. The nurses fascinating to look at, but their dress most un-practical,
entirely white from their veils to their shoes, & for walking, a voluminous,
well-cut, heavy cloth cape, reaching to the ankles. Apparently they do no
actual nursing, & have had but little training – even their Matron has only

done this sort of work since the war. The men apparently have shelter, a bed, medical attendance once a day, & sympathy – but it is not our idea of a hospital.

Having landed, [&] inspected the village & church, we wandered on to the camp where the French regulars are supposed to be. One officer came forward to speak to us & offered to show us round, but as he spoke *no* English & you know how much French we can manage, we had rather a funny time. When we came to his own Mess Tent, we were invited to have tea, & sat down to converse while we were waiting.... [He put] out his hand, asking were the Allies friends? I said certainly & gave him my hand – then we were each asked "pour un baiser" [a kiss], but on explaining that we were Canadians & didn't care for that sort of thing, he quite ignored his remark, was as polite as could be, & showed us the rest of the sights....

They have quite a number of Bulgarian & Turkish prisoners, but we were only permitted to view them from the wrong side of the barb-wire fence. Oh! & I forgot to mention the cemetery over there – over 800 British & several hundred French. Doesn't it seem dreadful, knowing how far we are from the actual battle field! especially as we have our own cemetery on this side besides. The demonstrative character of the French was even noticeable in their graveyard, so many of their graves having the most elaborate wreaths, beautiful flowers made of glass beads on wire, sent from Paris. Beautiful & yet hateful to me.

...

January 28th

Snatch[ed] breakfast in bed. At 10 a.m. got word we were to be at the Pier at 3 p.m. Everyone rushed out of bed & began to pack. Then I had to help in the Mess, but finally had to leave at 2.15 p.m. & so the men will just finish the best way they can. We had to walk down to the pier so had to allow a little extra time. We were fortunate in having a beautiful day, but as always it was a fearful rush in the end.

At the pier we had to wait about ¾ of an hour & then the lighter came & took us & our luggage to the Hospital Ship, "Dover Castle," just back from Imbros with 200 patients on board, & as they have room for 600, there is plenty of room for us. Our Officers & the unit, with the equipment, are supposed to join us to-morrow – but one never can be sure. Per usual we are in two large wards – but everything seems very nice & comfortable & you can't think what a treat it was to sit down once again at a decent look-ing table, with respectable china & etcs.

Well we're all off to bed early & I feel to-night ends one stage of this job. We may land in a worse place than Lemnos (perhaps!) but I feel mighty thankful to feel we have had this experience & are off the island none the worse for it. Well dear, I think I'll bring this letter to an end as it's pretty long, & start a fresh one to-morrow.

Heaps of love to you always from Lollie.

3

Alexandria and Cairo: Mosques and Minarets

The nurses of CSH No. 1 thankfully sailed for Egypt on January 31, 1916. They spent a short time in Alexandria before moving on to Cairo to rest and recuperate, staying at a nurses' home established in the stripped-down Semiramis Hotel on the banks of the Nile. Laura's letters demonstrate increasing irritation at the British authorities' lack of attention to the nurses' status as officers in the Canadian Army. The lack of equity for male and female Canadian officers in travel arrangements made by the British and the placing of the Canadian nurses under British regulations meant discomfort and unnecessary restrictions, highlighting the greater privileges, freedoms, and trust that nurses enjoyed under the Canadian administration. But Laura's and Mildred's letters also indicate the growing companionship they feel for their fellow Canadian nurses through their sympathy for Mabel Clint, hospitalized in Egypt, and their sightseeing expeditions with the other nurses.

Most importantly, Laura's and Mildred's letters illuminate nuances of attitudes towards what was, for them, an exotic and multicultural city. Both were to enter social work at the end of the war, and Laura would revolutionize Canadian social work policies for children and for women. On Lemnos, Laura saw the people she met – the villagers, the Egyptian labourers, and the French medical workers – as curiosities, noting their habits, especially those related to cleanliness and its lack. In Cairo, she went further, observing people, customs, and living conditions but also inquiring into the reasons for them. Her sympathies for women and children were honed by the gender inequities she increasingly observed in the military, including her experience of being treated as a "colonial" by the same British administration that had been indifferent towards its own soldiers in hospital on Lemnos.

Letter No. 42
S.S Dover Castle
January 31st, 1916

Dear Mother,

...

... I think I mentioned we got on board about 4 p.m. & immediately had afternoon tea, & were comfortably settled by dinner time. Have simply been revelling in the meals, which are mighty good & rather more like home cooking than is usual.

Rules for Nursing Sisters is off the deck at 9.30 so the evening isn't long, but I rarely find the time heavy on my hands anyway.... The one drawback to the boat is that there is no lounge room of any kind, & as the weather has been fearfully cold, one is either forced to keep moving on deck, or retire to the Ward & [lie] down on the bunk, for there isn't a tack to sit on. Needless to say the *officers* have a smoking room!

...

February 1st

Yesterday we sailed at 7 a.m. The wind blew, the waves rose & the boat rolled. I was forced to take to my couch, took a dose of Mothersills & by evening felt O.K – the wind in the meantime had gone down. Mildred had such a dreadful cold, & it was so miserable outside, we persuaded her to remain in bed. To-day is simply glorious – cool but not a bit cold, sun shining & the water a gorgeous blue. No excitements to report of any kind. In the afternoon, the Padre got up a concert, & the R.A.M.C. have some very good talent on board. In our own unit we have two privates with beautiful voices, one a baritone, the other tenor, but no one who can sing a comic or popular song of any description.

We arrived in the harbour (Alexandria) this morning ... & now are awaiting orders, hoping against hope to have some time on shore.... Love to Uncle & always your own self from Lollie.

Letter No. 43
February 3rd 1916
Cairo, Egypt

Dear Mother,

... Isn't it wonderful to think we are actually in Cairo, with every chance of remaining for ten days or two weeks? Of course there is a certain amount of un-certainty, consequently feel it wiser to go ahead & do all necessary shopping, for after five months in Lemnos our cotton uniforms are a sight; still we hope to do a good deal of sight-seeing as well. Being Nursing Sisters in uniform is an awful draw-back to thoroughly enjoy an outing, for it makes one frightfully conspicuous & we are more or less kept under rules & regulations – however we're mighty lucky to be here under any conditions.

Well to go back to yesterday (it seems at least a week ago) ... we reached Alexandria yesterday at 7 a.m. We thought our O.C. would have to go off & hunt up some official regarding orders, but to his & our immense surprise, we were expected, & when an M.T.O. came on board with definite orders, we all got a tremendous shock. [T]his is the first time since the unit left Canada that on arrival, [we] were even recognized but always had to inform headquarters who [we] were, wait while England was cabled, etc., etc.

Well the first order was to send the Sisters immediately to Cairo, where there is a large Nurses' Home. We were rather disgusted at the news, for our officers were not to come with us.... [O]nce separated one never knows what may happen, & none of us are keen to work in Imperial Hospitals. However we hoped for the best. Left Alexandria at 3 p.m. on a hospital train – & you would have died if you had seen us packed in on shelves, too many of us to allow for lying down comfortably, & yet most un-comfortable sitting on the edge, especially as Mildred & I had an upper bunk. The result was we stood looking out of the window most of the way. [A]lthough we were a good four hours on the way, didn't find the time long, for ... there was something of interest all the way.... The sight of green fields after Lemnos was almost bewildering – the numerous camels, weird looking cows & animals, the mud villages dotted here & there, & the great variety of natives was most fascinating.

The train had a few patients, & there was a very pretty V.A.D. on board, such an attractive English girl, who saw that we all had a very good & ... substantial afternoon tea. On arriving [at] the Home ... we got rather a pleasant surprise, for instead of a crowded dingy place where we all half expected to exist in Wards, we found a really palatial hotel, which the government have taken over as a sort of headquarters for Sisters in the Mediterranean Expedition. Uncle may know the place – Semiramis Hotel.[1] The drawing-rooms are closed, & all the etceteras done away with, the food is well cooked but badly served, & the rules while rather maddening really don't much matter.[2] We are perfectly free to go our own way all day but must be in & ready for our dinner at 8 p.m. [There are] numerous small rules, such as being always in correct uniform, not speaking to Officers, or going out with them at all. [T]he latter I consider absurd as one can go so few places without a man, & it seems absurd to trust us with any old drago-man in preference to an Officer we know.[3] However I feel sure our O.C. will permit us to go out with our own Officers when he arrives, & in the meantime as we know no one, it doesn't matter.

Mildred & I are together in quite a nice room, & oh! the joy to get right away from the crowd.

... [L]ast night we had dinner shortly after arriving. The waiters ... wear elongated white shirts reaching to the ankle, red shoes, red fez & red sash. It is most amusing to watch the head-waiter, in a grand silk gown of golden striped satin. We are supposed to all sit down to the minute, & no doubt if late for one course, miss it altogether, for when the grand individual consid-ers it time for us to have finished, our plates are removed, he rings a little bell, & every waiter flies from the room as though his life depended on it & returns with the next course. We had soup, fish, beef, tomatoes, cauliflower & potatoes, blancmange & prunes.

I believe the weather is un-usually cool even for Cairo at this time of year & certainly in this huge barren, dismantled building, we felt nearly frozen. There are no curtains, carpets, or fires – just an immense expanse of marble, hard-wood floors & tremendously high ceilings.

Breakfast this morning at 8 o'clock.... Then we did a little shopping but didn't accomplish much. Thought of going to Shepheard's Hotel for lunch, but on arriving inside didn't see a woman of any kind, suddenly felt shy & so came out! Then realizing we had to eat somewhere, for it was too late to go back to our own place, we came in to this hotel, where lunch was good but expensive.... [4]

My eyes just ache with looking at so much, & the sun seems much brighter than it has been in Lemnos for the past two months. Cairo seems so much cleaner & better class than Alexandria & the shops far more numerous.

... Rumour says our destination is to be British East Africa but there's no telling. We will probably know more in a few days. In the meantime we hear none of the hospitals are busy. Apparently there is little fighting going on, & this being the healthy season, few of the men are sick.

Au revoir for the present

    Always Yours lovingly
     Lollie.

Letter No. 44
Cairo
February 11th, 1916

Dear Mother.

... [W]e have spent endless hours in the shopping district, for while ... we have not bought a great deal, what we happened to need has been difficult to find. Naturally my greatest difficulty has been foot wear, & while the shoe shops are surprisingly good, suiting Canadians far better than the London shops, owing to the War ... no goods are being imported, & my size being rather an unusual one, everyone is out of it – if only I took ½ size smaller!! In desperation ... I ended by buying low black shoes – too large & fearful looking. However there are times when it is a great comfort to be able to change into something quickly. Now I have ordered a pair of tan boots to be made by a French shoe-maker & am hoping & praying they may be a success.

It is so difficult to know just what to buy, for everything here is so frightfully expensive, & should we be moved in the near future to either France or England, we could shop to so much better advantage – however just at present the betting is on the Suez Canal. I don't look forward to it in the least for the heat is terrible there after the middle of March.

In the meantime no one seems to be very busy – it is terrible to see such an immense number of our men doing practically nothing but loafing & yet undoubtably it is necessary for them to be on the spot.... Every day I spend here makes me marvel more & more that England has so much control here, but I imagine it's not held without effort. Of course Cairo is in anything but a normal state. The native part of it remains un-changed as always & [life] runs along in their quarter much the same as it has for hundreds of years, the lack of tourists un-doubtably adding to its charm – but the European quarter ... is very different. Shepheards is practically full of English Officers – just a sprinkling of guests in mufti[5] & an occasional female. The Savoy has been taken over entirely by the government for Officers, & the Semiramis for Nurses. The shops ... are ... doing a tremendous business, but the souvenir shops, perfumers, flower shops, etc. are doing nothing – one wonders how they ever manage to keep open. Numberless homes, especially of the rich, seem deserted – apparently several had to leave for political reasons & yet the place as a whole is anything but deserted....

... I have invested in a semi-silk sweater, a great convenience at times & in this climate almost a necessity. Mildred & I both feel many of the girls are mad on the subject of having numerous & rather swank uniforms, & far too extravagant – but I suppose everyone knows their own business best.

Personally I don't know how they manage, for I feel I am spending an immense amount, & yet every cent spent on sight-seeing ... is a good investment, for our stay is most un-certain, & such an opportunity may never come our way again.

Mildred & I are both investing in a blue tussore silk uniform for excessively hot days & in the hopes we may not be a disgrace to the unit when on board a steamer, for we are generally considered two of the shabbiest of the unit!! I must admit our cotton uniforms are sadly faded but there's good wear in them yet & why be too fussy in the desert? for once one gets to work what does it matter? The dress will cost when finished $13.50.... As a cotton uniform out here costs $7.50 I feel that isn't too bad....

...

February 4th

... In the afternoon we got a cab, Miss Hervey[6] & Kingston[7] joining us – drove to the Sultan's Palace to see the changing of the guards – not quite such an imposing sight as in London but still very interesting, & of course one never has enough eyes to see what is going on in a Cairo street. From there we went to the Caliphs Tombs [and] the Kait Bey Mosque.... [T]he first is I think the gem of any I have seen so far. From there we drove to the Citadel, where the magnificent Maehemet Ali Mosque[8] is – but I can't attempt to describe any of them until I get home for they are so numerous & all different. The view from here you have heard Uncle describe so I won't repeat – but it certainly is true that nothing about Cairo can be exaggerated.

The weather is perfect, beautifully cool in the shade, & this time of year comfortably hot in the sun, almost cold at night; the sun-sets are gorgeous, the people fascinating, the filth & dirt beyond description, & the whole place teems with interest. My one regret is that I know so little of its history. After leaving the Citadel we went through two more Mosques ... & then as it was getting quite dusk, thought it wiser to go right to the quarter we knew, so drove & had tea at Groppi's & then walked home, just comfortably having time to dress for dinner. Groppi's is the popular tea-shop where they have luscious cakes & candies, & good tea & coffee.

February 5th

We had made arrangements with nine others to go down the Nile to Barrage. Started at 9.30 a.m. having hired a felucca manned by two natives, neither of whom spoke English. As there was little wind the men were forced to row a large part of the way & we reached Barrage about 1.30, having previously eaten a picnic lunch in the boat.... We all thoroughly enjoyed the sail (?) but it is not an ideal way to go, for being so low in the water, one has practically no view, the bank of the river being higher ... & the land so flat.

The gardens at Barrage are wonderful & we were fortunate in having the Curator ... [show] us around. The Barrage, by the way, is one of the large dams for regulating the height of the Nile.... [A] large amount of the surrounding land has been cultivated, & the result is this beautiful park. It is really a little early to see things at their best, the trees are all still very faded & dusty looking, but some of the flowers are beautiful. Around the grounds on the outskirts there is a little railway, with the queerest cars, pulled by natives, & on these we rode to the station, a distance of about two miles, & came back by tram. At every station one is besieged by beggars, noise & confusion.

...

Well Mildred is in bed & sound asleep, & as I am good & ready myself think I will say goodnight & continue in the a.m.

...

Always love from Lollie.

Letter No. 45[9]
Cairo
February 12th, 1916.

Dear Mother,

... It is so difficult to realize that you are in the midst of probably miserable winter weather, whereas this climate at present is perfect, so beautifully cool that unless one is right on the desert with the sun streaming down, a cloth dress feels quite comfortable, & in the evening a wrap a necessity.

Well to go back to Monday the 7th.... [W]e took the train as far as Mena House where we all (four) got on camels to go to the pyramids. We had great fun, & once on their backs quite enjoyed the sensation. I was not disappointed in the least in the pyramids, but one can't help regretting the Sphinx is so surrounded by clamouring photographers & numerous children yelling for "bacsheesh" – one gets to hate it. I won't attempt to describe any of it except that the desert even for me, hating the sun as I do, has a wonderful fascination. The coloring in the distance, the inevitable camel in the foreground, & the rolling sand in all directions is lovely. We just sat down on a heap of sand & enjoyed our lunch (you feel very luxurious always having a boy trailing on behind carrying your lunch) & a smoke & then

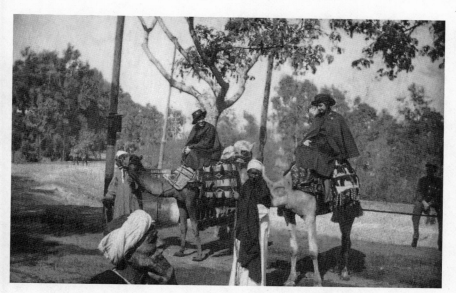

Laura and Mildred on camels, Egypt 1916. *George Metcalf Archival Collection, Canadian War Museum, CWM 19790413-012_p27e*

decided it was too expensive work loitering, so wandered on our way, the guide taking us through the Bazaars. Of course I could spend hours & hours wandering there, not so much on account of the goods displayed as to watch the people at work, so many using the most primitive implements. I have made up my mind to buy nothing, for I have seen nothing you would like specially ... & it is so doubtful when we will turn homeward that I think it foolish. Sometimes I have weak moments & wonder if I am making a mistake, & then the future seems so un-certain ... that so far I have managed to stick to my original resolution. Our guide apparently has taken numberless good customers through & so is greeted enthusiastically by many of the vendors without our ever being pestered to buy.

On Tuesday the 8th the morning was again wasted in the shops. Although I say wasted, I really enjoy every minute I spend on the street, & am afraid it is largely owing to this I loiter so much & accomplish but little. Had a shampoo in the afternoon. Unfortunately most of the hair-dressers are French, consequently are at the front, so while I got a good shampoo, the curl was miserable. Wandered into Groppi's for tea, then went for a walk.

Wednesday 9th shopped in morning again & went to the Egyptian Museum in the afternoon. A wonderful place, although at present everything is up-set.... Came back to the Hotel for tea when we un-fortunately ran into two men we had met, & felt obliged to be polite to – consequently when they left it was too late to do anything.

Thursday 10th. We had a wonderful [day].... We hired a boat (there were over 30 of us – mostly Sisters, a few Officers & a guide...) & went up the Nile, a gorgeous trip. Had lunch & arrived at our destination about 1.30 p.m. Here we were met by numerous donkeys & rode in all 7 ½ miles to Memphis & Sakkara, through two small villages, farmland, & then the desert. We only had time to visit two of the excavated Temples, but the trip from beginning to end was full of interest, & coming back the setting sun going down behind palm trees with those wonderful green fields in the foreground beyond description. The donkeys were a surprise to all of us, for in Lemnos they are sure-footed but terribly slow – one can scarcely ever get them to run – whereas here one can't get them to stop. My poor little beast became tired on the return trip & although it still persisted in running, twice its knees gave way & I was sent flying over his head, fortunately landing in the sand, so none the worse. You can imagine the spectacle! Mildred also was unfortunate, her donkey treating her the same way. We got back to the boat at dusk....

Friday 11th. Woke up to find I was bruised from head to foot but felt the day had been well worth it. This morning we took the train to Heliopolis, a magnificent suburb of Cairo, with numerous beautiful modern buildings but nothing historically interesting. We wandered around, & had thought of driving out to the Obelisk similar to the one in London I believe, & the only antique in Heliopolis, but the cabby persisted in charging us double fare so we got mad & wouldn't pay it. When there is so much to see for less it wasn't worth it.

In Cairo itself one never has any trouble for there is a tariff but apparently not at Heliopolis. In the afternoon treated ourselves to tea at Shepheards, where there is an orchestra, but were disappointed it played so little. I must say had I un-limited means & were visiting here in the proper season, I should much prefer the Savoy or Semiramis to Shepheards. The situation of the Semiramis is simply perfect, right over-looking the Nile & surrounded by beautiful private residences.

To-day (Saturday) we again were extravagant & had a guide, our nice man, & decided to go alone, for one can do things so much more quickly when several people have not to be consulted. We went first to Old Cairo, where we saw the oldest Mosque in Cairo, the wealthiest Synagogue, & an old Coptic Church now in the possession of the Greek Priests. At this latter church we were fortunate in running in when service was on. It seems hard to believe that their teaching is nearer ours than the R[oman] C[atholic].

Uncle will tell you about Old Cairo, its poverty & filth. I simply can't describe the abject poverty, families living in tumble-down houses, where the sun has shone for hundreds of years, the floor mud, & the entire furniture ... one wooden bench, one bowl & a water jug. Why they don't die I can't understand. I asked the guide how much rent one particularly old woman he spoke to would pay – & he said she had inherited it from her husband & so had neither taxes or rent. She was a Christian, & like all members of the Coptic Church, had the Coptic Cross ... tattooed ... on her wrist.

From there we went into a very old Coptic Church, built over the spot where the Virgin, Joseph & Christ were supposed to have lived during the time they spent in Egypt. Just at present this Church is beginning renovat[ions] – the remaining bits of in-laid work are exquisite.

...

From here we visited another old Mosque ... popularly known as the blue Mosque as it has such wonderful blue tiles. Here, since England has taken Egypt in hand, free schools have been established as well as in many other old Mosques, & it is curious to see the children squatting around in groups, a teacher sitting on a bench tailor-fashion, reading out something or other, the children repeating it with him. A few yards further is another group. The noise & confusion is immense, & one can't help but wonder if any of them really learn anything....

...

Each day I think it is more wonderful to be here, seeing & learning so much. There is still no news of what we are going to do. Au revoir for the present & heaps of love always from Lollie.

Letter No. 46
Cairo
February 14th, 1916

Dear Mother,

When the mail arrived to-day I more than got a shock on finding I was the recipient of *12* letters, but on opening them the shock was even greater for they all dated back to October!! ... In one way it is frightfully disappointing, on the other I am awfully glad to get them all, even at this late date.... Also received ... a box of eatables sent in September!!!! Sometimes I regret anyone having sent anything, & yet it was just the extras from home that made life as comfortable for the last three months on Lemnos ... & the thought of having so much now in our boxes takes away all terror of arriving again in some god-forsaken place. After all in comparison to what we received not a great deal has been lost. Of course the birthday box is the big one. Every time I think of it I feel heartsick. I know just how much work & money it represents – & then when I remember how we all got away from Lemnos in such good health, & safe & sound, I feel one has no right to grumble.

Of course when I read Mrs [F.'s] letters, telling me what *heroes* we all are, I feel ashamed, for while of course the first three months in Lemnos the discomforts were awful – after all in the end, we did not suffer, & now we are having a most wonderful time here, under no expense & ... in comfort. Really isn't it wonderful! especially feeling we are not surrounded by suffering. At times it hardly seems right to be enjoying ourselves so much & yet it would be foolish not to make the most of such a wonderful opportunity. You don't know what I would give just to have a good old talk with you; somehow when one sits down to write it's so different.

...

    Always love dear – I only wish I could talk to you as often as I think of you—

    As ever, Lollie

[P.S.] ...

Letter No. 48
Cairo
February 19th, 1916

Dear Mother,

    ... [O]ur dresses ... have ... come home, & look very well, though the silk is too thin to look smart in a plain uniform. However they are beautifully cool & that is the main point....

    I think I mentioned getting a silk sweater, but in reality it is a mercerised one. Your daughter & Mildred are the two plain common-sense women of the unit. As far as possible we are saving our money – I feel there is every chance of our needing it after the war, for times are bound to be hard, & if not will save it towards a trip. Some of the girls have simply gone crazy over the shops, I think – buying the daintiest of underwear, silk kimonos, etc. Isn't it absurd on active service? I suppose it's sort of a reaction. Don't read this out to anyone, for it only arouses criticism & what's the use, for after all they are not half so good to themselves as most of the Officers.

    Of course I think we would be silly to miss seeing the sights – but otherwise until we know when we are going home, or what the out-come is to be, we can't be too careful.

February 16th

... In the afternoon we went to the Anglo Egyptian Hospital to see "Clint,"[10] one of our Sisters who has been miserable for some time, finally has developed what appears to be a very bad phlebitis – as we couldn't attend to her properly here, she was sent to this hospital & is to be transferred to England as soon as they are able to move her. Poor girl, I feel awfully sorry for her. She is far from young – intensely interested in her work, & being of an active disposition, is going to find it difficult to live the life of an invalid – for everyone seems to think it will be months before she will be able to work again....

February 17th

...

... [W]e went through various lanes & by-ways & came to an old Egyptian house, which is quite well preserved & was most interesting, giving one a capital idea of the plan of a Mohammedan's house. The woodwork & mosaics were lovely. Certainly from a man's point of view, the eastern ideas are perfect. From here we again visited Kait Bey Mosque.... Finished up by visiting a little out of the way mosque, where we went up on the roof & watched the boy ... go out on the minaret & call the people to pray. Many of their ideas are beautiful, but in this more modern world, some of the ceremonies lose their point & this seems to be one of them, for although in olden times apparently *everyone* when called to prayer went, now very few seem to respond. There are many fanatics & good Mohammedans, but compared to the population, one can't help but feel there are many who are lukewarm....
...

Love always from a rather weary
Lollie.

Letter No. 48
Cairo.
February 24th, 1916

Dear Mother,

... Everything points to Salonika, in fact the O.C. says short of having a *written* order to that effect, that is where we are told to prepare for – & while it isn't positive, only something un-foreseen means anywhere else. In many ways I'm glad it is not to be Egypt, for I would dread the heat, & at least Salonika is farther north, though they say none too cool. Conditions they say are a second Lemnos – supplies short but by now they must have necessities....

The O.C. is delighted at the possibility of getting to Greece, & from a professional stand point thinks it a great opportunity, & I must say to be where the work is, is the only thing that makes being here worthwhile, for I hate the life ... in a hospital when there is nothing doing. There is no use saying too much about it, for of course it is not a certainty. One thing, we won't have to pave the way as at Lemnos, & being near a town of sorts there must be water in plenty, which is the chief thing.

The day before yesterday, on the spur of the moment we decided to go for a ride on the desert, something we had often wanted to do. Miss Hervey (rather more of an old maid than we are), a quiet rather congenial soul, joined us; we got a guide & went out back of the pyramids.... [I]t was one of the loveliest trips we have had. The shadows on the sand as the sun goes down [are] wonderful, & there is just a something in the very atmosphere, once out on the desert, that is fascinating, but entirely lost when with a crowd. It was quite dark when we got back to the train, & we had a great rush to get back on time for our eight o'clock dinner.

Yesterday we wandered through a large garden ... just across the Nile. You would love the huge rubber trees, for their leaves are so bright & shiny. Poinsettias varying from eight to twelve feet high, covered with blossoms, but we arrived too late apparently for the leaves. It is so difficult to follow the seasons here for I imagine some plants bloom continuously, others only at certain seasons.

...

Love to Uncle George, & always for yourself.
As ever Yours lovingly
Lollie.

[P.S.] ...

Letter No. 49
Cairo
February 29th, 1916

Dear Mother,

...

Life drifts along very pleasantly, though we are now taking the days a little more quietly, for even without the heat, one can't keep on the go continually in this climate....

The poverty to me is frightful, & always in one's line of vision. While one knows the goods of this world are not divided as fairly as they should be – here it really worries me.... [S]omehow even away out here one feels the world is topsy-turvy, & it is impossible to feel one is on a pleasure trip, even if there is no work at the moment to be done....

...

Love always from Lollie.

4

Salonika:
In the Shadow of Olympus

B etween 1430 and 1912, Salonika was ruled by the Ottoman Empire; in
1912, it became part of Greece when Serbia, Montenegro, Bulgaria, and
Greece joined forces to defeat the Ottoman Empire and strip it of "al-
most all of its European territories."[1] When the First World War broke out,
Greece suffered a severe political crisis: King Constantine, married to the
Kaiser's sister, sympathized with Germany; the prime minister, Eleutherios
Venizelos, was sympathetic to the Allies.[2] During the Dardanelles campaign,
Venizelos offered Salonika to the Allies as a landing place for troops, which
infuriated King Constantine.

In the fall of 1915, Bulgaria allied with Germany, declaring war on Serbia
in October.[3] Although the Allied forces attempted to protect Serbia from
attack, they arrived too late, and the Serbians were forced to undertake an
arduous retreat through the Albanian mountains. The British and French
governments then decided that a campaign in the Balkans might provide an
alternative means to victory; this new campaign became a "permanent fixture
for the rest of the war."[4] By the end of 1915, approximately 160,000 British
troops were stationed around Salonika.[5] However, the disagreements between
King Constantine and the Allies resulted in instability in the city, and on June
3, 1916, French troops "imposed martial law" on Salonika,[6] as Laura documents in one of her letters home.

Laura's letters hint of preparations for an attack in the summer of 1916, and
some action did take place in August and September,[7] with more in April
1917. The main offensive did not take place until the summer and fall of

1918, when the Allies finally overcame the Bulgarian Army, forcing Bulgaria's surrender on September 29, 1918.[8] Salonika was "a forgettable campaign" that cost the Allies more casualties from disease than from the fighting.[9]

Laura and Mildred again found themselves nursing mostly medical patients instead of wounded, albeit the men "came in much less depressed than the men from Gallipoli."[10] CSH No. 1 treated mostly men with enteric diseases and malaria. Malaria was rampant due to the swampy, mosquito-infested terrain, and the "sickness rate" was "so high from the summer of 1916 onwards that the hospitals were choked."[11] CSH No. 1 admitted 658 patients in June, a figure that more than doubled in July and August.[12] Malaria was "prevalent" among the medical staff, and a steady stream of unit personnel were invalided to Malta or England, including Matron Charleson.[13]

For the rest of the war, the CAMC nurses of CSH No. 1 would compare their new postings to Lemnos. Salonika posed its own challenges, but for Laura, Mildred, and their fellow nurses, a good water supply and sufficient medical equipment seemed luxuries to be thankful for. Regular time off, too, gave them the leisure to better observe the vibrant multicultural atmosphere of the Greek city, where British, French, Serbian, and other soldiers mingled on the streets, and to try to alleviate the difficult circumstances faced by the refugees they encountered.

> Letter No. 51
> R.M.S. "Lanfranc."
> March 2nd, 1916

Dear Mother,

You can imagine our surprise on boarding this boat to hear we were once again to see the little isle [Lemnos] we had left such a short time ago, & never expected to be near again. And in just these few short weeks it is hardly recognizable. The points, which some months ago were a mass of tents & thickly populated ... [are] now a picture of peaceful pasture land, with soft patches here & there of a mossy green. It looks ideal & yet I've no desire to land.

...

We got word in the afternoon [of Sunday, February 27] that we were to leave the following morning by the 9.30 train, & got off quite comfortably – & am glad to say this time we were allowed to travel 1st Class, & not on shelves as previously! One doesn't mind in the least putting up with any hard-ships or un-comfortableness that is necessary, but it does make one inwardly rage to see the way the English government give the best they've got to any *Officer* from a 2nd Lieutenant up – but grudge it, even if it's no extra expense, to a Nursing Sister. Certainly once [a woman] steps out of her own home circle, an Englishman seems to think [she] should receive no consideration whatever. Of course in his own family it's different.

We arrived at Alexandria about 12.45 noon. Drove over in motor ambulances to the boat, & went on board immediately. I had hoped to have had time to send you a cable, but was not allowed ....

...

We did not sail until 6 p.m. so had time to get comfortably settled. And certainly, the feeling on the boat has never been nicer. There are absolutely no rules or regulations. The Matron of the boat has been so nice & hospitable – & apparently the O.C. of the boat has made the officers feel the same way, & the privates of the unit say they have never been so well fed or more comfortable since leaving Canada....

For the first time on any hospital ship we have seen, there is a lounge room for the Nursing Sisters, which is really a general lounge room. Previously the one & only place off the decks was reserved for the officers, & we weren't allowed to put our noses in....

...

... We expect to leave here in an hour & to arrive at our destination in the early morning....

March 3rd

Very rough last night. Felt pretty sick but O.K. this morning. Port just in sight, & letters are to be landed immediately, so au revoir for now.

Always Your lovingly
Lollie.

Letter No. 49
H. S. Lanfranc, Salonika
March 5th, 1916

Dear Mother,

...

The entrance to Salonika is truly lovely. I wish I could give you an idea of what a picture it [is]. The city, a mass of softly tinted square buildings, closely clustered together on the side of a hill, topped by a most picturesque citadel or fort, around which runs an ancient city wall, evidently in almost perfect condition, & owing to its situation can be distinctly seen. Numerous minarets, similar in shape, rise up here & there, & against all these soft pastel colors, one sees an occasional dark cypress tree in the background. The buildings run right down to the water's edge, in the distance everything so neat & tidy, it reminds one of a model. On either side rise the most beautiful hills, here & there soft patches of green relieve the brown tones, but no trees. On the opposite side of the harbour rise a whole line of snow-topped mountains. It is beautiful!

So far we have not been allowed on shore, but the Officers who have been through the town on business say it is appalling – the filth of Egypt is nothing by comparison. Isn't it curious, for even from our boat, which is tied up to the wharf, the city rising gradually in front of us is a picture! However there is not much chance of our spending a great deal of time in the town's midst, for one needs numerous escorts, passes. etc., for it is guarded & picketed at every corner.... I was very surprised to find so many mosques, in my ignorance not realizing this country belonged to the Turks for ages, & only was restored to Greece after the Balkan War.

The Camp is about four miles from the town I hear, though the distance seems to be somewhat of an open question.

We are taking over a New Zealand Hospital['s] ... site, & I believe the two O.C.'s have made one or two little exchanges. [F]or instance, we're taking over *some* of their tents.... The work promises to be disappointing, unless the un-foreseen happens, & our stay more or less of a limited one. However as you know, one never can tell what may happen, our life depends so much on the movements of others. But oh! the colossal waste of war – it's positively depressing.

Our hospital now owns a motor ambulance of its own, & this is going to be a tremendous help, especially during our first week or so.

...

We're mighty lucky to be here, for I'm sure the climate is much more promising than the Suez or Persian Gulf – & so long as we're right out of the town, it's bound to be healthy. Love to Uncle George & yourself. Yours in the best of spirits,

Lollie.

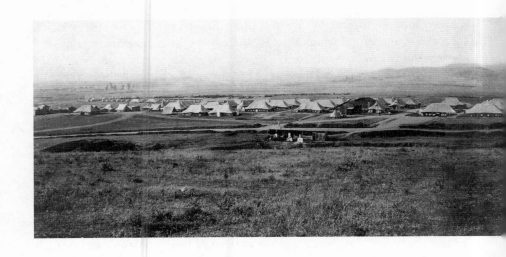

Letter No. 52
Salonika.
March 8th, 1916

Dear Mother,

I'm not a bit in the humor for writing, but know you'll be looking for a line, so thought I would just say hello!

The same old difficulty of not knowing just how much we are allowed to mention arises – but so far I always seem to have kept within the limits, so shall still chance it I think.

The usual under-current of dissatisfaction (usually in connection with work of course) is always more apparent during moves ... & things are somewhat at boiling point. [B]ut it's useless to discuss it & most un-wise to say the least – but it's not conducive to a peaceful, happy-letter-writing mood. They are not so much personal things, as kicks against the little pricks of the whole system of military hospital ways. The only way to look at it is that in spite of the many mistakes, in the long run an immense amount of good is really done, & one can't help but feel *now* is not the time to raise a hue & cry, but just dig in & do the little one is permitted to, in the best way [one] can.

I've been talked *at* & *to* so much this a.m. my head is in a bit of a whirl, & I must get away from the subject.

...

It seems so dreadful to be sitting down doing nothing, when the privates are working themselves to death – & yet to interfere or suggest there *are*

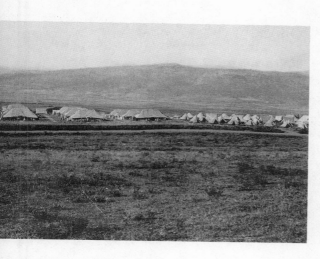

Lembet Camp, Salonika, 1916. *George Metcalf Archival Collection, Canadian War Museum, CWM 20070103-014_p48*

things we are quite capable of doing would be breaking military regulations & creating a furore. Most of these little difficulties arise or rather fail to be over-come owing to one thing only, & that can't be mentioned, but I'll have to explain a good many things to you when I get home & am once again free to express my own opinion. [I]n the meantime I wouldn't – for worlds.

Our comparatively new O.C. is most energetic & business-like & will in time overcome most of our difficulties, at least so far as is in his power. I like him very much.

We are *all* in tents. [W]ith the exception of a small wooden hut for the X-ray department & the corrugated iron latrines, there is not a building on the grounds, but the weather promises to be good, & under those conditions it must be healthy.

There are only four in our marquee – Mildred, a Miss Harman (M.G.H),[14] funnily enough an old St. Georg-ite in Toronto, her family still being members of Uncle Bob's congregation. She takes rather a blue out-look on life but is a very nice girl & splendid room-mate. Her friend Miss Kingston, another Toronto girl, is the fourth. She is rather an old-maidish, *very* lady-like girl – deadly, but quiet, & also a splendid room-mate. It really is far more satisfactory to have the entertaining & hilarious ones in someone else's tent – to go & enjoy when so inclined, & have your own quiet spot to return to when sick of the row.[15]

I can't give you any idea of our surroundings – we're too much in the midst of things for that – except to say it's rolling country, high hills quite close, *no* trees, but more grass & less roughness than on Lemnos. We are ... about four miles from town, food I think will be much easier to get, & once the hospital is in running order, ordnance store & Red Cross, I rather imagine, much more plentiful & easier to get than where we were before.

...[M]y few lines have lengthened into many, & still I have not mentioned what I started out with first in my mind – & that is your Xmas cake, the cigarettes & candies ... arrived yesterday! Isn't that fairly good time? Of course [they] really went to Alexandria, but ... [weren't] distributed until we reached here – but ... couldn't have come at a more welcome time.... When I think of all you have done & are doing, I simply gasp, for I know how the house duties have to go on just the same. It seems to me the people at home do far more than we do.

...

       Ever yours lovingly,
       Lollie.

                                      Letter No. 53
                                          Salonika
                                  March 11th, 1916

Dear Mother,

     Mildred has just written you a long epistle, I know – but on the chance that no two people write quite the same way, think I'll send a few lines.

     I feel sure Mildred must have told you what an idle week we've had – & we are still told there is no work for us to do. There are a few convalescents, but evidently we are not needed, & as you know in this life one has to do as they are told!! Thursday ... hearing there was a chance of going into town on the ambulance, Mildred & I jumped at the opportunity; once in town, ... not being allowed to separate from the others, as the O.C. insists on an Officer being with us ... we saw little except the main shopping street. There is little chance of our having to do without necessities here as in Lemnos, for one can get anything in reason, although the prices are exorbitant! Huntley & Palmers biscuits, $1.30 for a two lb. box, & many other things accordingly.... [A] few prices are not out of the way. Eggs I think 50 & 60 cents a dozen. But it means a great deal to feel things *can* be got.

     On the way in, instead of feeling we were on a country road, the traffic was as bad as on St Catherine Street,[16] but these are the details one can't enlarge upon – except I suppose we may mention that we passed numerous low brick buildings, built in the time of the Balkan War for the Turkish refugees, now being used for Serbians. Poor souls, four walls is about all they're given, & I suppose daily government rations. After the war is over, there will be a wonderful lot of work to be done educating these children to some trade, [&] finding employment for all these idle people. The whole out-look is over-whelming – but I suppose in time things will right themselves.

...

March 16th, 1916

... [W]e've been on duty!!!! We may not have been needed, but ye gods! it would have made our work much easier had we been on a few days sooner, for men are men, & don't do their work the way a woman does, & of course our orderlies are un-trained, & no matter how willing, aren't capable of arranging things convenient for nursing. Then you can imagine the dirt. Everyone has been rushed to death ... un-packing, & something had to go, but it seems to me it would have simplified matters to have had us on. However in this life one is not supposed to have any ideas on any subject.

...

... We went on duty Monday morning, & while we only have about 200 patients in all, have had to keep at it pretty steadily, trying to arrange the tents & work conveniently, & we're a long way from being settled yet. To begin with all the tents have been "mudded" to make them fit in with the landscape. I can't understand ... just why [we] have to make ourselves inconspicuous as regards tents, when they have to go to all the trouble of making two immense red-crosses on the ground in order that aeroplanes may *see* we are a hospital. Then each tent, even when crowded, can only hold 16 patients. This means so much running, for in a district where there is a possibility of an air raid, the space between must be large for fear of fire, & so we can't string the tents to-gether as in Lemnos.

The hospital is divided into Lines, each line having five tents, four of which have 16 patients each, the middle one only eight, as half of the tent is used as a Service tent; here we keep the dressings, food, dishes, etc. When I tell you there are ten to twelve feet between each tent, you can imagine how much running about we have to do. It's most inconvenient, but of course we are not permitted to do any of the arranging. Certainly this is a place where a woman seems to show much more common-sense than the general man. He can't grasp the difficulty of getting food around.... However perhaps when everything is in running order, it may work out better....

...

So far only three out of five boxes we had sent from Lemnos have turned up.... The ones we opened seemed to be principally from Mildred's friends

– you can't think what a help they have [been] the past few days. Oh, conditions here are nothing to when we landed in Lemnos. Of course with ... equipment like we have, after six months active service, nursing is rather up-hill work.... [O]ne can't make things convenient in this life, & living & working in tents that are always pitched in a hurry ... is not comfort, *but* we have the necessaries – there is water, light of a kind, far better food, & so far less work. I don't feel it's hopeless at all, as we did before, & while we may have to run round in circles un-necessarily, still I feel the patients we have are being looked after. Their food is fairly nourishing – even the air seems healthier – & certainly they came in feeling much less depressed than the men from Gallipoli, so altogether the out-look isn't too bad.

...

> Ever Yours lovingly
> Lollie.

> Salonika
> March 11th, 1916

My dear Cairine,

...

In our various moves I have lost some of my things among which was your letter telling me what the Rockland Red Cross were doing for us.... I have an idea you said that you were sending over money to London for the Red X there to ship us supplies. I got an invoice from them saying some cases were being sent & they did not mention the donors. The cases contained soldiers' comforts, 50 lbs. biscuits, tinned milk, & lime juice & lemon squash. Well, three cases have reached me containing the lime juice, lemon squash & biscuits. The others have yet to turn up. I wish I knew definitely if they were from you. The biscuits are splendid, put up in hermetically sealed boxes, and the "drinks" are awfully good, & very much appreciated, as every drop of water we drink must be boiled & the addition of the fruit juices makes all the difference in the world....

...

Well – here we are back in camp once more, and at present are far from busy. We are only too thankful to feel our troops don't need our care, but it is a monotonous existence sitting about in tents doing nothing.

We are rather crowded in our tents, but hope later on our huts will be put up, & I will be thankful to have a floor under me once more.

We had two soaking wet days this week, & spent our time trying to keep our possessions dry, for the tents are not rain-proof entirely. One gets a very damp cold feeling living under canvas.

This country is very attractive – it is very hilly, & snowcapped Mountains are in the distance. We can see Mt. Olympus quite clearly. I wish I could remember all Miss Smith had endeavored to teach me in Mythology & Greek History.[17]

The soil is much better than that of Lemnos – no rocks – & the earth is a rich reddish brown. Everything is getting green (not the trees for there are none in sight), & flowers are cropping up. Such lovely little crocus & bright colored flowers totally unlike any I have ever seen.

The camps about us and various activities are interesting – we feel we are nearer the war than we have been yet. The doings in the air are wonderful, & I only hope they may not prove exciting for us!

We went into Salonika the other day in an ambulance – one feels it would be a very interesting place, if one were at liberty to wander about ad. lib. We were pleased to see that the shops were quite fair, & that we will be able to purchase necessities (at an exorbitant price unfortunately.) However we are well supplied, thanks to you.

I hope my next letter may be more interesting, but on account of censorship it is difficult to write.

Hoping you are all well, and with much love.

 Affect. yours.
  Mildred H. Forbes.

Letter No. 54
Salonika
March 22nd, 1916

Dear Mother,

...

Time simply flies these days, & while we're not specially busy, somehow settling & trying to get things in running order is rather worrying work, & at night being four in a tent is not conducive to letter writing. I do so hate *never* being alone for one moment, for even in one's time off someone else is there too. I know when night comes I just tumble into bed, try to read, but never can settle to anything else. They are putting up our old Lemnos canvas huts, & in spite of their being in a terribly dilapidated condition ... I shall be delighted to get in one, just to feel we have one corner to call our own. Previously each sister had her own hut, but now there are to be two – it will be frightfully crowded, but can't be helped.

...

... We've spent the week scouring, & trying, with the help of packing boxes ... to make the place look rather tidier & more convenient. It's up-hill work for we have to wander round the grounds & swipe any packing case we happen to see around & quite often get called down for taking one that is not supposed to be touched. It's really rather amusing, for one feels it's scarcely a nurse's duty, but no one else seems to consider it theirs, & so we do the best we can. However it has been heaps easier than at Lemnos. To begin with there is plenty of water, better food – in fact more of everything, & of course our boxes have been a perfect boon. Mildred has received seven more from some chapter Mrs. Wilson is interested in, & with the others [they] have meant more than I can say.

It would have done your heart good had you seen the pleasure some of the things gave to fifteen men, all well enough to go straight back to the trenches. They happened to belong to the same unit, & most of them had been through some pretty bad fighting in France, were amongst those who made that awful landing at Anzac,[18] & afterward were in the retreat in Serbia, where they said they had the worst time of all. Doesn't it seem hard after being lucky enough to come through so much to have to go back to the firing line? for the Sergeant Major told me, once firing began, they would be sure to be sent right in it. Such splendid men – & there aren't any too many of the real Tommies left.

Well, for their last dinner, as I happened to un-pack the box that contained your Xmas pudding, I gave it to them, for I felt no one would appreciate it more, & they more than enjoyed it with a good stiff brandy sauce. I was able to give them all an extra pair of socks, a pack of cards each, a pipe, tobacco & cigarettes, & some chocolate.... [T]hey left, I know, with very kindly feelings towards Canadians. I only wish you all who have worked so hard to get all these things together could see how much pleasure they are giving. Although the Red Cross supplies, I hear, are wonderful in this part of the country, so far we haven't had a chance to get hold of them, & anyway, I doubt if we ever get quite the same sort of things.... I was quite disappointed not to have some of your pudding, for no one makes them quite the same, but felt these men deserved it more. Our patients on the whole are such splendid men, much nicer than those we had on Lemnos, more cheerful, & not nearly so sick & miserable.

We are rather tied to the Camp, & can go *no-where* without an Officer, & even then must not go out alone with him – but the surroundings really give one a splendid idea of the running of affairs at a time like the present. Of actual news we get practically none.... Much Love Always Lollie.

Letter No. 55
Salonika
March 29th, 1916

Dear Mother,

Imagine our surprise yesterday, on opening one of the boxes ... to find it was my birthday box.[19] Isn't it great to think it has finally turned up! I'm simply tickled to death, & thanks to you being such a wonderful packer, everything arrived in splendid condition – the candy ... hasn't that delicious creamy texture [as] when eaten fresh, but age has failed to spoil its flavor. Robinson's cake was quite damp – I could hardly believe it. The biscuits are great to have, for once our stock here is finished, we can buy no more for the prices are awful – don't take this as a hint for more!!! ... I feel our time here is so un-certain, it would be foolish to send anything more, especially as we can get a good deal in other lines.

... I wish you could see our tent, we simply can't move. I have cases at the foot of my bed, at its head, & by the side, two full ones make our wash-stand! But oh! the joy of having them. Mildred had a patient who died to-day, & his brother came down yesterday from somewhere in the trenches, & his gratitude for a few odds & ends made one feel quite "weep-y" ....

Mildred has received a large number of boxes also, & every one has contained such useful things. One parcel with a few extra heavy bed-socks made out of eider-down were too heavy for this climate ... also a few heavy scarves, [so] we took [them] up to a few tumble-down cottages where dozens of families huddled together, Roumanian refugees, & their delight on being presented with these things was pathetic. Such intelligent bright looking kiddies, one longs to take them away from this poverty & idleness & give them a start somewhere & a chance to earn their living or rather learn how to do so. They all wear such wonderful costumes ...; no doubt in their own country they were fairly well to do peasantry. Everything is hand woven – none of the materials apparently bought – even to their aprons being heavy homespun, every color in the rainbow mixed in together, forming either plaids or stripes.... My! but it's a draw-back not being able to speak to any of these people. We were invited in to have "coffee" but to my regret we had to refuse, for it is strictly against rules & regulations.... All villages are considered out of bounds also.

...

When I start in thanking people for all they've done I do feel so helpless, for nothing I can say seems to give any idea of what all their thought & trouble has meant to us & the men. The latter of course don't realize quite as we do what an immense amount of work it means to make & get together all these articles, but they appreciate it as much as any *mere* man can. Certainly you take the prize for packing – as well as getting through an astonishing amount of work – but then you always were a wonder.

...

... [H]ad a very interesting little trip two days ago, & saw the result of activities over-head – the destruction possible is terrible – but can't go into details.[20] There is no fear of my forgetting them. I[t] seems awful to say so, but even these tragedies have their funny side – & during the excitement the other day, the costumes around our camp at 5 o'clock in the morning were killing.... [21] Heaps of love dear – I can never thank you enough.

> As ever Lollie

> Salonika
> March 29th, 1916

My dear Cairine,

I have so much to thank you for.... [T]wo days after writing my last to you, I received some boxes from the Canadian Red Cross in London containing splendid supplies, & I feel sure that it is the Red Cross of Rockland who are responsible. Thank you all so much, for the things are beautiful & arrived in very good shape. We got khaki shirts, handkerchiefs, games, cocoa, books – & all are being made good use of & are so much appreciated.

Although our supplies are much better here than in Lemnos, yet we are so thankful (Lollie & I) to have a private supply to draw on, & it makes work so much easier to have these things – & if you could see the pleasure the men get out of them. It is splendid to have the things to give them. Everyone has been so kind in sending us things & I feel badly that I have so little time to write & thank them. But these days I am rather busy – & tired when off duty. ("Things" seems a favorite word.)

If I could only tell you of the excitement we have from time to time, & I only hope we will all get home intact![22] But it is no use worrying. We must all "play the game."

This climate (about the only safe thing to mention) is at present delightful, though I hear malaria is apt to be prevalent later on. It is a nasty thing to get but cannot beat dysentery, which we had to fight before.

Well I have so many letters to write, I must close now. Excuse scrawl – with much love & Many thanks. Aff. Yrs. M.H. Forbes.

Salonika
April 19th, 1916

My dear Cairine,

By the time this reaches you I expect Rockland will be looking lovely, with all the trees out and your garden "coming on." How I wish I could pay you a visit – [t]hough we would never get to bed at night for I would have so much to say!!

Today I received from the Can. Red Cross ... a box of Condensed Milk – a most appreciated donation. I wonder if it, too, is from Rockland. You have been so awfully good about sending us things, and if your Red Cross were to stop work right off, you could feel you had made one lot of people very happy.

I have your letter of March 9th which came a short time ago. The tales of snow storms certainly seemed curious in this country, though the nights here are decidedly chilly. We are very glad of our coal oil heater in our hut at night. It must be an unhealthy climate for as soon as the sun goes down it gets so chilly. The days are not too warm yet, though I always am on duty & out of doors in a cotton dress & no sweater.

...

We had a day in town yesterday. It was quite a whirl for us, & we both feel quite exhausted today. It is the first trip for over five weeks, so you see we do not lead a dissipated life.

The morning was spent at the hairdressers where Lollie got a wonderfully good shampoo & wave. The surroundings would have amused you, but the man worked well & was clean.

We had lunch at a Restaurant where the service is awful – food pretty bad – but the best place in town. Then after some shopping we went to a Band Concert on the "Front." It is lovely along the Harbour. There is quite a wide street & one can walk along quite close to the water. It is all interesting, but the sidewalks & roads are so rough – cobble stones – that we were exhausted after a short walk.

It is an interesting town, full of all nationalities, but such dirt & confusion everywhere.

It is hard to realize that Easter will soon be here – life is so different with us that we feel adrift from all ordinary life, & I cannot think that everyone at home is still going on in very much the usual way.

I suppose once we go home this experience will seem like a dream – however I feel sure it is bound to change us. My disposition (never of the best) is ruined. Army life is one too much for me.

Well, I must close now & get ready to go back on duty.

With much love to you all

    Affect. Yours.
    Mildred H Forbes

                            Letter No. 60
                                Salonika
                           April 28th, 1916

Dear Mother,

Miss Hervey, who put in sometime ago her resignation, has received orders to be prepared to be transported to England at any time, & so on the chance that she may leave in a day or two, thought I would send you a line via England, & for once avoid the Censor.

As far as our little worries & troubles in the unit go, I wouldn't go into them for the world. All that will keep until I return, for it's far wiser to mention no names. I wonder once we get away from it all if the little pettinesses that show so prominently now, will then seem as bad.

At times one feels the number who are out to do their bit the best way they can are so few that their influence can't be felt at all. So many are after what they can get out [of] it one becomes disgusted! However, we live such a narrow life & our out-look is so limited that this partly accounts for it. Mind you I am not speaking of our own unit only, although I by no mean[s] exclude them. Well here's hoping anyway, that next fall will see the end of the war, & all our present trouble.

We have just had three solid days of rain, the tents are all fearfully dirty, [and] our clothes are muddy, none of which lends to a cheerful atmosphere…. [T]o add to it all I have a pain under my pinny – but no doubt to-morrow the sun will shine & all will be well. On the whole we have had wonderfully fine weather so have no right to grumble, & even now the wind can't begin to compare with the wind of Lemnos after two hours rain.

I wonder if it is worthwhile describing the day we went up to see the trenches – I know you are interested anyways.... The ambulance left about 2 p.m. taking ... five sisters & two officers.... We had not more than an hour's run, practically all up-hill, passing various camps & field ambulances.... The car stopped at the top of the hill, we walked a few yards further & look[ed] out on such a wonderful plain, all cultivated, the whole looking like a checker board, each square representing ... a field of oats, barley or some grain, each one a different green, the monotony here & there being broken by a bare square, showing the richest of brown earth. At three different points squatted ... three small villages, each looking most diminutive & toy-like, [which] must have housed the farmers for all this land – then beyond rose more hills, behind which the enemy is supposed to be in possession. I think I am right in saying Bulgaria can be seen in the distance on a clear day. To the extreme right one can see Lake Langaza,[23] ... about five miles distan[t], & one straight white line shows the only road leading to the enemy's lines. It is just this plain that makes our position so strong, for they say the enemy could never cross it, our side being so well fortified.

At this point the M.O. of a certain division met us, & we were taken through the 3rd line of trenches, now un-occupied. In front, at the foot of the hill, could be seen the 1st & 2nd line of trenches, but time would not allow us to walk that far, so we stayed at the top of the hill. Of course I can't describe the immense amount of work these preparations demand. Mile after mile of trenches, many parts of which are entirely concealed by placing sacking over-head & throwing small shrubs & a little dirt on top. Then the observation dug outs,[24] with branches of trees in front to conceal the windows, etc., the same where the guns are hidden. It was most interesting. None of the large guns are on the brow of the hill, but placed at a slightly lower level on the downward grade at the back. [T]he man in the observation dug out sends word by phone in what direction the gun is to fire, & so they fire according to his command. Doesn't it seem wonderful, that the gunner is in a dug-out & only the muzzle of the gun is un-protected! I can't decently explain it, although since actually seeing the positions, understand it.

Then we went still further down the protected side of the hill & came to the Officers' & mens' dug-outs. Really they were wonderfully comfortable under the circumstances, although the men are pretty well fed up with their monotonous existence. The O.C. had a very nice tea ready for us. Potted meat sandwiches, biscuits, tea, served of course in enamel cups.[25] Except ...

for the monotony & the un-certainty of the future, they are not to be pitied, for as far as comforts go, they have far more than we do – I mean of course better food, more servants, etc. ... [N]aturally it won't be quite the same if any active work commences. But to me it does seem that there is far too much difference between the way Officers & their men are looked after. Often the latter don't get bare necessities where their Officers are having all kinds of luxuries, & naturally this doesn't lend to the contentment. However I suppose it always has been so & always will be, but I feel sure if there ever is another war during our life time, that they never will get the number of men necessary to volunteer again – it will be conscription or failure.

...

I wish I could give you some idea of the surrounding camps. They are on all sides of us.... Unfortunately there are numerous artillery camps, which means an immense number of horses, a very bad thing to have anywhere near a hospital, especially in a country where flies are so numerous anyway. However I don't quite see how it could be avoided....

Although the two Canadian General Hospitals are only a few miles distant, I have never seen them. It means arranging a special trip, & not knowing any of them personally, don't quite like to wander in.... However would rather like to see how they run their places. One is the Toronto Unit, No. 4 General, the other the B.C. Unit, No. 5 General.[26]

No. 3 Stationary who were with us on Lemnos & No. 5 Stationary who were in Cairo have both gone to France, we hear.[27] Our people are most envious! Personally I'm not anxious for another up-heaval just at present.

...

... Good night & heaps of love always. From Yours as ever
   Lollie.

Letter No. 61
Salonika
May 1st, 1916.

Dear Mother,

... Mildred tells me she has written you quite a long letter in her time off, but just thought I would add a few lines, as Miss Hervey has word to leave on Wednesday, & I hate to miss such an opportunity. I can't tell you how sorry I am she is leaving.... I think I mentioned before she is on my line & what I will do without her I can't imagine. It is not only that she is a splendid worker, but [she] seems to have so much influence over everyone around her. Her patients are always contented no matter what goes wrong, the orderlies like her – & not being young & flighty, one doesn't have to worry over her hours off. Oh! well the break had to come, & I can only hope some-one fairly decent will come in her place. At present so many of the girls are off duty sick that I doubt if I get anyone! ...

...

... [M]y time off to-day has been entirely spoilt. First when I came off found a man visiting our camp that I had met before, & *had* to do the polite [and] get him tea.... Then immediately after dinner, went to a committee meeting to discuss Mess matters. Our troubles in this line are too complicated to discuss in writing, but every day I put up a little prayer of thankfulness that I am not Mess President, who so far has also been Mess Sister – that is the girl who does the buying, manages the orderlies, & regularly has the devil's own time of it, for the powers that be don't help her out in any way.[28]

...

To think I never mentioned the *Cake*!! had arrived. You can't think how we're enjoying it. The parcel arrived in perfect condition ... & before I even got the cake out of the box, by the aid of a knife, Mildred & I managed to get a big slice, & we sat & feasted & had our fill on the spot. It seemed such ages since we had had a bite of cake. Phone Nora & tell her how delighted I am – but I simply haven't the energy to write her to-night.

I seem to have grumbled so much in these letters home, am afraid you'll think I'm un-happy. Mind you, I won't be sorry to get home, but under the circumstances it's not too bad, & it's such a relief to say what one feels like, knowing it won't be read by a member of this unit! As far as I can make out every unit has its own little worries & troubles – I think it's living in such close quarters, & having so little variety. One is scarcely ever alone, & night after night one just comes off duty & goes to bed – you know for certain people this is fatal & a general air of discontent reigns. Well I *must* stop. Heaps of love dear always

   from Lollie.

             Letter No. 62
               Salonika
            May 7th, 1916

Dear Mother,

Nearly a week has gone by since my last.... I can scarcely believe it. Just tell all my friends the heat is arriving so not to expect any more letters!!! I don't really think it is any hotter to-day than a warm day at home in August, but with no trees in sight, & living under canvas, one doesn't seem able to get away from the heat of the sun. However suppose it is nothing to what we may expect a little later on, though perhaps by that time we may be on our way to England. One thing, I don't find it nearly so trying as I used to. I know I'm going to feel the cold dreadfully when I come home – but with our warm, comfortable houses, it won't matter what the weather is outside.

Well last week altogether we had quite an interesting time in comparison to the usual monotony.... [W]e saw a German taube, brought down some distance from here two days previously. As it was not badly damaged, expect it will be patched up & used again by our people. They are so different from the French aeroplanes.... The latter are typical of what we have seen in England & at home.

[On] Wednesday night ... our A.S.C. man ... asked Mildred & I to go to a concert, which was being given by a motor transport unit. As he has a very comfortable motor, & the concert was held on the other side of Salonika, the ride itself was a treat. The programme I enclose & it really was capital. There were just seven men, dressed in black pierrot costumes, for the chor-uses, & a few special ones for character songs.... Afterward we had sand-wiches, lemonade & *cake* in their Mess Tent, & then drove home, having thoroughly enjoyed the outing.... Of course these concerts are put on chiefly for the benefit of the surrounding camps, & give an immense amount of pleasure, & they always manage to get remarkably good talent. Then not to have too dull a time, we had another raid on Thursday night. I was sleeping like a top when I heard our O.C. shouting through our lines there was a Zeppelin overhead, & to get to our dug-out.[29] Dead with sleep, I managed to find my kimona (no lights allowed), & with Mildred tore for the dugout. As a matter of fact the Zeppelin wasn't near us, but the anti-aircraft shot was over-head & that is really what the O.C. is afraid of. I can't tell you what a wonderful sight it is, seeing the magnificent search lights all focussed on the one object, & every shot from the anti-air craft guns illuminating the sky. It's a sight not to be forgotten quickly – and then to think it (the Zepp) was brought down without having done any damage. Am wondering if there will be any objection to our mentioning this, but as it is all in the paper, can't see that it matters.

...

Well my hand is simply sticking to the paper – so guess I will stop. Always love dear. Truly wish we could have a good old talk. However some day –

Bestest love As ever from
  Lollie.
[P.S.] ...

Dear Mother,

...

    This is the first really cool day we have had in some time, so feel rather more energetic than usual; unfortunately there is a Wesleyan service on in the recreation tent at 1.30 p.m., & nobody to play the hymns, so expect it's up to me, as I am off duty to-day from 1 to 4 p.m. We always manage to get three hours a day off, either from 1 to 4 or from 4.30 for the rest of the day, & really I don't think we could stand it otherwise.... As it is, there always seem to be two or three of the Sisters on the sick list, & that means a Sister to look after them; so far I've been fortunate since arriving here, & so has Mildred.
...

    I don't think I wrote you about our trip last Sunday. It was such a nice change. A friend arranged a nice little trip in a motor-boat, sending out his motor to call for us.... You can't imagine what a treat it always is to get right away from the camp & its surroundings.... We went out to try & see the Zeppelin that was brought down early in the month, but as it fell on very marshy ground, practically out in the sea, & surrounded by very shallow water, we couldn't get within half a mile of it. The men had brough[t] such a nice afternoon tea with them, & having a primus stove, we were able to boil water ... without ever slowing down a bit. Spent three hours on the water & got back just in time for our 6.30 dinner, feeling we had had a delightful outing.

    I can't imagine anything lovelier than Salonika from the harbour, with its back-ground of hills.

    On our day off we decided to spend the time in town, as I wanted a hair-wash badly – our quarter-master came with us, being one of those good-natured men, always willing to take one anywhere they feel so inclined. Unfortunately none of us are allowed to stay in Salonika for lunch unless accompanied by an Officer & on no account can stay in for dinner, so one usually has to plan ahead....

... [I]t was after twelve before my old Greek had finished my shampoo. I must admit his results are good – but oh my his methods are slow, & as he can't speak a word of English, neither can he make anything of my French, it is impossible to make any suggestions or remonstrate in anyway.

...

Having heard there was a small exhibition of paintings being shown for the benefit of the Red Cross, thought we might as well have a look at them after lunch. The exhibitors are all French men – the majority I imagine just in the ranks – but all celebrated & well-known ... in their own country. There were about 200 pictures & sketches – all more or less local subjects & needless to say most interesting – whether valuable or good from a technical point of view I don't know enough to say. All were roughly framed in narrow plain wooden frames – the wall had all been hung with plain khaki material – so the effect was quite gallery-ish. Doesn't it seem wonderful, at such a time & under such circumstances, that such an attempt should be made? But that is the French for you – they are so energetic & ingenious, & no doubt it is just this interest & keen[n]ess that makes them all appear such a happy lot. The difference between the two armies is so noticeable; the French, as a whole, perhaps a cleaner looking lot of men, but much more slovenly, never uniform, having little appearance of discipline, just a happy-go-lucky, cheerful lot of men – who however in regard to their work accomplish wonders. You would laugh to see the numerous & varied uniforms.

...

We have met several Officers who are fortunate in owning cars for their work – but the rules & regulations are mighty strict, & they are not allowed to carry any women as passengers, nurses or otherwise. Occasionally we have taken a chance & trusted to luck, but not often, for they are the ones to get into trouble & not ourselves. It does seem rather mean [that] our one chance of a little variety should be taken from us – but that is the disadvantage of being a woman. It seems rather mean when we are forced to put up with all the disadvantages of this life that they are, & yet cannot indulge in the few privileges that they are able to take advantage of. However this I suppose is war! or the vileness of men....

...

The fly problem is our greatest difficulty at the moment. I found a tempting dish that killed them by the hundreds, until my service tent floor was a mass of carcasses – but it seems hopeless, for with the tent always open, fresh ones fly in as fast as the inmates die, & when viewed in such masses ... a dead fly is almost more nauseating than a live one.

...

Goodbye for now. Always love to you
    from Lollie.

Salonika
May 29th, 1916

My dear Cairine,

...

You are so good about writing, and I appreciate hearing from you so much. I realize how busy you always are, and when night comes it is an effort to write – I know I find it so. My one idea is to go to bed & read, & [I] nearly always fall asleep.

I have just discovered to my horror that April 19th was my last to you. I am sorry I have been so remiss, but I have written very few letters from here, as one seems able to tell so little.

We have had some hot weather, but nothing to what we will get in July & August. The flies are out in full force. They are simply disgusting, [and] they also will increase with the heat. Altogether it is not a pleasant prospect. As long as we can keep well, it won't matter much about our discomforts. I feel we may be more or less immune from the diseases prevailing. Surely our taste of an Eastern hot season will assist us this year. There is a lot of dysentery around, due to sanitation and the water. We of course boil every drop we use, but I fear other camps are not as careful.

Our Hospital has been full. Last week was a busy one. We receive patients from the various field ambulances every other week. We alternate with the other Hospital in receiving patients from this [place], but we take in Men from the various outlying Camps anytime, so we keep busy always, especially in the Medical Wards.

Lollie & I are both confronted with night duty. We go on next week for two weeks. It is a necessary evil and I shall be glad to get it over before the worst heat. In a way I shall be glad of a change – I have been in charge of a line for nearly three months, and although the responsibility is not great, yet there are lots of small worries & fights. This life is enough to ruin one's disposition. The Army is an extraordinary concern to be in, and I think women find it more irksome than men. People tell me that one should not have a conscience, and certainly we come in contact with many who have none.

On our afternoons off we have gone into town, for there is always something of interest to see there, and we get so "fed up" with the camp, and driving in on the ambulance is at least cooler than sitting about here. The bazaars there are interesting – there are lots of things to buy, antique and modern, but I often feel unless one is a connoisseur one is apt to buy something made in Birmingham or Grand Rapids, Michigan. I have bought nothing, for we seem to have so much junk to carry when we travel and so often these things when taken home are useless.

...

This country is really beautiful, but I will be glad to see the last of it. Last night we had the most gorgeous sunset. Lollie & I went up on a hill and watched the sun going down. The lights on Olympus were wonderful. The Harbour was also a sight.

I wonder if you will all get to St Andrews. How I would love to join you! Well I must say goodbye, and with Much love to all.

Affectionately Yours.
Mildred H Forbes.

Letter No. 66
Salonika
May 31st, 1916

Dear Mother,

We have just heard that three of our number who have not been particularly well lately have been invalided home, & will in all probability leave sometime to-morrow, so thought I would drop you a few lines, for one feels a little free-er to gossip, knowing our particular Censor will have nothing to do with it....

...

Merriman & Cook, both nice girls who are being invalided home, are supposed to have rather weak hearts, & the O.C. thinks they will not pick up in this climate. Bell has some kidney condition, & the necessary diet cannot be had here. We all feel very badly, for quite apart from liking them all personally, the whole three are splendid workers, & will be very much missed on the Lines. We are short-handed as it is, & I dread to think of the predicted rush. However it may never come off.

The troops continue to move up the line, & one can hardly believe so much preparation can be going on without it resulting in some active work. Of course on the other hand their position may be so assured [that] there will be no occasion to fight. It is curious to listen to the conflicting rumours. Colonels ... visit us from various points away up the line, & each one, in

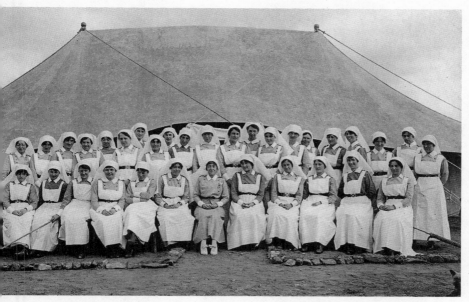

Nursing staff, Canadian Stationary Hospital No. 1, Salonika, 1916. *Back Row:* Bell,
Helen Fowlds, Laura Holland, Mildred Forbes, Myra Goodeve, Turner, Scoble,
Brock, McCullough, Smith, Hammel, Lloyd, Rogers, Hunter, Brown, Kingstone,
Drysdale, Clarke, Upton, Bertha Merriman, Johnston. *Front row:* Bruce, Juliet
Pelletier, Blewett, MacNaughton, Jones, Fray, Matron Charleson, Cooke, Harman,
Kidd, Meiklejohn, Didion. *George Metcalf Archival Collection, Canadian War
Museum, CWM 20070103-014_LPb*

spite of being right in the midst of affairs, differs as to what is going to
be done....

As to our own unit, it is hopeless in a letter to go into the state of affairs
at all, except to say we're all fed up – but then so is everybody else.... [A]s far
as I am personally concerned, think we're mighty lucky to be where we are,
for there is plenty of work (for the Sisters in particular), we have the satisfaction of feeling we are doing something, & I know I'm far happier under the
circumstances than I would be had I stayed at home, though I admit, no one
will be more thankful than I will when I hear peace has been declared & we
can pick up stakes & go home. But a move to France has no charms for me,
or in fact a move at all. However there are all kinds of rumours hovering
around, so that one feels far from settled, & in spite of being practically in
rags, I hesitate to send to England for clothes, hoping I can last out until I
can go & buy things myself.

...

I do hope you won't feel I am at all unhappy, for I don't mind the life in the least, & the dis-comfort is [small] when one realizes how much more the majority are enduring.... [T]he reason I think one gets so fed up is that on all sides ... there seems so much un-fairness & neglect of duty going on, causing so much trouble for others, that one is inclined to rant & rave & feel "all's wrong with the world," & perhaps forget to notice the many who are in for the good of the cause, & doing their bit the best way they can. But there is no doubt War conditions don't by any means bring out the best in one, except in those who are left at home.

... [W]e continue to have gorgeous weather. Too hot for camp life, but ideal if one were leading an ordinary life, living in decent quarters with the usual comforts of life. Last night ... Mildred & I ... went ... to the top of a hill nearby, from where we could see the harbour in the distance & the surrounding country. The sun-sets are wonderful, & with Mt. Olympus in the distance, a grand sight. [O]ne never tires of it.

...

 Always Yours lovingly
 Lollie

P.S. Forgot to mention we have been told, if we dread the heat we can go ... [to] England on three months leave – needless to say as I feel perfectly well, haven't the slightest intention of asking for it, as we are needed here, & feel sure I can stand the conditions as well as the next one. Have no idea how many will take advantage of the opportunity, & only hope re-inforcements will be sent to take their places.

Letter No. 68
Salonika
June 4th, 1916

Dear Mother

To-day we had rather a wonderful afternoon, quite un-expectedly, & no doubt on that account all the more enjoyable.... [W]e ... thought we would try & get a glimpse of ... [Salonika] itself, under present conditions.... [O]n the 3rd (yesterday) the Greeks were celebrating their King's birthday, when in the midst of the demonstration, the French calmly walked in & took possession of the town, which is now under martial law. No resistance was shown & the whole affair was settled quite quietly. We expected to have some trouble getting in, general orders having been issued that no British officers were to go in except on important business. [H]owever we took a chance & were not stopped. The town looked much as usual, except that few people were about, no Greek soldiers except those on the quay waiting for a ship to take them ... dear knows where, but anyway out of Salonika. At every corner a French soldier stood with bayonet drawn, guards were everywhere to be seen, & the more important buildings had extra guards on duty. Every soldier obviously had his full equipment with him – rifles & pistols seemed very much to the fore.... [But] the stores were open, [&] we went as usual & had tea.... [W]omen were conspicuous by their absence, & very few English Officers were to be seen, all evidently remaining in Camp in case of trouble.

It was rather one on us that while we were having tea, our most senior officer ... sat at the table next us & inquired if we had not received orders to stay in Camp. I replied yes – but that we couldn't starve & we had come in on *important* Mess business! He laughed & said "Oh! I guess it's alright – as far as I'm concerned I haven't even seen you"!! So – I guess it's alright. On our way back we ran a few miles down the road to see the remains of a large fire we had noticed burning in the distance the night previously. It was several thousand tons of fodder belonging to the A.S.C., set [on] fire by a Greek I believe, who[m] they were fortunate in catching. Poor man, I suppose he'll be shot.

...

On our way home we ran into a whole battalion of Scotch men, headed by the inevitable bagpipes, here & there the stretcher bearers, & in the rear the pack-mules carrying the field guns. Such a magnificent lot of men, all in their kilts & khaki aprons, everyone dusty, dirty & tired, with the per-spiration just pouring down their faces, but the majority cheerful, several batches in spite of the heat having energy to sing a popular song or two. We ran into them just by the Serbian refugees' huts, & there were several hun-dred of [the refugees] lining the road, making a brilliant picture in their red & startling orange colored aprons, a few here & there having quite magnifi-cent metal ornaments on their heads & around their waists. It's impossible to give you an idea of the whole picture – one gets so many impressions, [&] everyone you pass is interesting. I came back feeling I had had one of the most interesting afternoons I have had since coming out here, & at the same time a most enjoyable one. It is now mid-night, & time for me to make rounds so shall have to stop.

...

Before closing I must mention the Serbians. To my surprise somehow, they are such magnificent men – most noticeably so. Good-looking, well

built, & the cleanest & best groomed men around here, the British not
excepted – really it's wonderful; as someone remarked, only the fittest have
survived, [so] perhaps that may account for it.

...

> Always love dear from
> Lollie.

Letter No. 69
Salonika
June 8th, 1916

Dear Mother,

...

Now that I am on night duty ... I haven't energy to want to go anywhere.
Not but what I am feeling well, but it is hard to sleep comfortably now it
is so warm, & one gets up feeling like a rag. Once on duty however, it is
perfectly cool & comfortable & I'm ready for anything. The first three nights
I was awfully busy but things have quieted down now. Came on duty last
Sunday night & so have just a week & one day more. Did I tell you I was
now on a surgical line? Really a change does one good. The surgical patients
are so much brighter & more cheerful than those in the medical lines. The
latter, poor souls, are usually half dead when they come in, whereas a man
who has had an accident is in perfect health.

...

Have I ever mentioned [that] Miss McCullough,[30] who is now our Mess
Sister, has been just as good as Upton & her successor, Miss Scoble?[31] We
really have been most fortunate. [T]he girls in turn have worked so hard &
been so interested that our meals are really excellent. I can tell you after those
few weeks on Lemnos with *nothing* fit to eat, we appreciate all good things
to eat, & realize how important it is to have nourishing food. But how I'd
hate the job myself! Miss McCullough is the type who gets on famously
with men – is good-looking, stylish, has nice clothes [&] silk stockings ... &
everyone is anxious to help her, so her buying has been most successful. But
food is a villainous price, & worse than ever since the blockade. However
we're being paid good salaries & so can afford it.

Lately we have had a little trouble in the line of Greek children prowling
around & stealing. Our huts are on the outside line of the hospital grounds,
& ... we are the people who have suffered most. In consequence we have had
a good barbed wire fence put around the place to-day. In the morning the

O.C. caught four wee children in the lines – tied them all together & put them in the dug-out for an hour. Then one of the men who speaks their language came & talked to them, & warned them they would be severely punished if found stealing. Poor souls, none of them were over ten – & they had had nothing to eat since the previous morning. So they were given a meal ... & sent off. And there are hundreds of others like them.

I know as early as 4 a.m. one sees many of them walking over the hills – heaven knows where they have come from or where they are going. Each garbage heap they pass is picked over & any possible food rescued. No wonder they steal anything they can lay their hands on. I wonder what will become of these people when they grow up – one can't expect much from them.

What a shock the death of [Kitchener] must have been to everyone. Somehow one never even thought of such a catastrophe. One regrets he didn't at least live until peace was declared – & yet I can't help but feel he did his greatest work, & saw its result in one sense. It may sound curious, but un-doubtably it has affected everyone here far less than had we been at home. I notice it so amongst the men, all of whom admire him tremendously & were they at home would feel dreadfully; but somehow the majority have been through so much & had so many surprises that nothing upsets them unless it is bad news from their own families.
....

  Ever yours lovingly
  Lollie.

Letter No. 70
Salonika
June 13th, 1916

Dear Mother,

Well the girls finally got off to-day, & with them went my letters, so hope you will receive them ahead of this.... Six of the girls went & needless to say we are going to miss them very much indeed – some of them personally, & all in the work. There was Smith, Johnson, Cook, Merriman, Donkin, & Bell. Am awfully sorry Donkin has gone, for she [has] a very common-sense, rather sweet disposition – I like her very much. Cook, Merriman, & Bell were really *sent* home on account of their health; the others while invalided to England in one sense, have gone really for a change & rest. We were ... all given the privilege, but much as I hate the heat, guess I can stand it as well as the rest. The past few days it has been 100 ... in the shade, & as there is very little of that, you can imagine what it is like in the sun! At 6.30 p.m. yesterday it was 106 in the sun. However marvelous to relate, so far it has not made me feel at all sick or headachey. Of course sleeping during the day in a tent is almost impossible, but I've only four more nights, & really don't feel done out at all. Of course we're getting good food, which helps a whole heap, & my appetite is A.1. When I think of Lemnos, I feel we have a whole heap to be thankful for, though ... the hospital itself is much less convenient, making the work ... unnecessarily hard. However, I suppose it's not for me to criticise.

...

We are having wonderful moonlight nights, a great comfort – the nights are not nearly so cool as at Lemnos. I seldom have to put on my sweater. Dawn begins to break at 3 a.m. & it is quite light at 4 a.m., so as far as the night is concerned it is rather nice – the one objection is trying to sleep in the heat.

By the way we have just had a tin bath given to the Sisters' quarters, & a special ... corrugated iron bath house has been built to put it in. So far no water has been attached, but we have to get a man to carry it some distance in pails. Perhaps they may be able to attach a rubber pipe in some way – otherwise if we get a bath a week, we'll be lucky. I've had one, & oh! the relief to have more than an enamel basin to wash in, though the latter seemed a luxury after those canvas affairs we had on Lemnos.

...

Well I'm dead sleepy & will have to move round. Love to ... yourself always from

Lollie.

Salonika
June 22nd, 1916

My dear Cairine,

As I am seated in the hairdresser's waiting for Lollie, who is having her hair washed, thought I would make use of my time. The process is a lengthy one, & as I don't like leaving L. alone, & also don't care about wandering about the streets by myself, I have to sit & wait.

The heat has been terrific lately. Really I don't know how we are going to exist. It has been up to 107° [F].[32] As soon as the sun rises the heat is unbearable – at six a.m. one is boiled & so it goes. The tents & huts are awful & there is no place to go to get into the shade.

One mercy is we can get a limited supply of ice, so can get cool drinks. But one longs for a cool plastered house & some shade (& baths!).

I came off night duty a couple of days ago, thankful that my two week term was over. The nights were nice enough to work in, but the days were awful – sleeping was out of the question. Life drags on very monotonously. To be off duty is a misery for one feels the heat even more when not busy.

Today being our afternoon [off] we decided to come into town by the 2 p.m. car, & most of our time will be spent at the hairdresser's. However it makes a change getting away from camp. The road in is always interesting, crowded with all kinds of transports & all nationalities.

The air in town is not very salubrious – there is always a queer smell – which is to me associated with the East. It is a mixture of filth & spices.

I wonder if you are at St Andrews now. Oh, for one of the lovely breezes!

What we will be like by September I cannot imagine – all melted away I expect.

Excuse the scrawl. I have no news & am too hot to think.

Much love to you all.
Mildred.

Letter No. 71
Salonika
June 24th, 1916

Dear Mother,

For the first time in three weeks I feel absolutely normal. [C]ertainly night duty does not agree with me, & trying to sleep during the heat is a night-mare; however, thank goodness I've had my share for some time to come. The heat has been pretty bad the past three weeks – never a cloud, the temperature varying from 95 to 107 [F][33] in the shade, & not specially dry heat at that. I can't help but marvel how well I feel, for although I hate it & fairly exist from day to day, it does not make me feel sick as in the old days.

Am afraid my letters will be very short for some time to come. If one is off duty from noon until 3 p.m., the flies are so troublesome & one feels so hot & sticky, nothing is accomplished; & if on duty from 8 till 4.30, you are so tired that [you] flop in a chair on the shady side of the hut & stay there until bed-time. No wonder people become lazy in such a climate! However I know you will understand & not mind – & the rest of the family will only get an occasional post card.

I came off night-duty last Sunday morning, so slept until noon, then got our good-natured quarter-master to come to town with [me], for I wanted to get my hair washed, & the little hair-dresser being next to anything but a respectable-looking hotel, wouldn't dare go alone. We went in by the 2 p.m. ambulance, but found to my surprise the place was closed – so he must be a Christian. [T]he majority of the shop people close on Saturday but are open on Sunday. However was glad I went in, for we found a nice cool corner down in some Tea Gardens by the White Tower, where there was a beautiful breeze blowing off the sea ... & I really felt comfortable for the first time in two weeks. The boats & people always are most interesting – the place itself far from attractive, food poor, & prices exorbitant! but oh! the coolness, & to get under a little shade. Really town is much cooler than the Camp, & our quarters rather in a hollow, & therefore the hottest part of it – however it might be worse.

... Mildred & I got off yesterday, & went to town again – in fact we have made up our minds to go in on every opportunity for one can get a *cold* drink or ice-cream, & it's a change & cooler once you get there, & such a relief to get away from here. This time I did get my hair done, & while the heat of that stuffy little shop was beyond words, it was worth it. My one regret is Mildred had to suffer at the same time – un-fortunately there is only one basin & one man, so we can't both be done at the same time. However she managed to get two letters written so her time wasn't alto-gether wasted....

I still continue to marvel at the wonderfully good-looking, well-groomed Serbians. They are the most fascinating looking lot of men I have ever seen, & at present their number seems legion.

...

Well good night & good bye. Don't be disappointed if for the next two months you get only a few lines. I'll try & send them regularly so you'll know we are well at any rate. Mildred has gone as assistant in the operating room, much to her disgust, for while in one sense the work is easy, she dis-likes the work, and hours off duty ... are un-certain & can't be depended on.

I am on a surgical line, & do practically nothing but dressings. I'm not crazy about surgery as some of the girls are, but like the line I am on & the girls I am working with very much, & oh! the relief not to be running a line, & having to look after the supplies & food! So in spite of the heat, I am feeling particularly happy, so there is no need to worry.

...

Yours lovingly
Lollie.

Salonika
July 3rd, 1916

My dear Cairine,

I am picturing you seated on the verandah at St. Andrews, getting that lovely air. I am seated in my hut, with flies buzzing around me, in a melting condition. We are counting the days till September when we are promised cooler weather & some rain – until then life is a burden.

We tried celebrating the 1st of July. The men of the Unit had a baseball game, playing some of the men from the Toronto Unit (No. 4 General) which is situated about six miles away. Then we had a concert in the evening. The performers were the few in our unit who are accomplished, unfortunately a small number. Lollie was a good deal to the fore, accompanying the singers & playing herself (much against her inclination). We have had a tent with stage put up in a hollow, so that the audience sit on the rising ground. [I]t makes quite an amphitheatre, and reminds one of the old Greek days. Who knows that this same spot was not used for the same purpose many years ago!

I think the type of performance has rather deteriorated since then! Quite a few outsiders came and we had a light supper in our Mess tent, where the men out-numbered the girls 25 to 1.

We are extremely busy these days – there are so many cases of sickness at present. The heat is fearfully trying for the troops.

I am in the O.R. at present, a place I don't enjoy particularly. Our work there is not hard, but irregular. A good many night cases, and it is disappointing when one has planned on a cool peaceful evening to find the programme suddenly changed.

...

I have thought of Rockland so much, & told Lollie of the lovely trips we have had on the river, and the lilies of the valley coming out, etc. etc. It all seems so far off, & I feel as if I had always been in this life. It will be a happy day when it is all over.

There is no news at all. Everywhere I look just now I see horses & *mules*. The latter are used a great deal. We have a Veterinary Camp quite close, so there are always lots of horses there. The mules are brought down to be watered by the stream, which is just about 50 yards away from us. They are wretched animals & so stubborn. [I]t is funny to watch their antics – one man with four mules has his hands full.

Much love to you all & hoping the summer will be a good one.

Affectionately Yrs.
Mildred H. Forbes

Letter No. 72
Salonika
July 5th, 1916

Dear Mother,

It's over 100° [F] in my hut, with scarcely a breath of air but do want to send you a few lines to let you know both Mildred & I are O.K. You never would recognise your daughter these days, running about in the blazing sun, & being none the worse for it. Of course we all have lost a few pounds of flesh & I get an occasional headache, & while one can't enjoy [oneself] in this intense heat, it's wonderful to feel as well as I do – & marvelous to relate my appetite [is] good....

Did I tell you we were now getting a limited amount of ice? You can't imagine what a blessing even the little we have is. Unfortunately no ice-boxes of any kind have been provided for the hospital, so up to the present haven't been able to make the most of it, but gradually we are getting the patients interested & improvising a box out of packing cases, lined with tin-biscuit boxes, surround[ed] with excelsior, & then covering the whole with a blanket. Curious to relate, such details are always left ... to the Sisters, when one might reasonably expect some member of the unit would provide something for all the lines. However one has to accept conditions as they are & do the best [one] can under the circumstances.

The hospital has every bed filled & will continue, I imagine, to be busy so long as this weather lasts. The average temperature of the patients is abnormally high, 104 to 106 [F][34] – on each line a daily occurrence for numerous patients, & quite frequently an odd one higher. This means ... frequent spongings, & so long as there is no active fighting & no wounded, one can cope with it. I presume under different circumstances, they would be shipped immediately to the base. Our line is really a surgical one, but we have been forced to turn half of it ... into a medical one.... I've seen more *bad* peritonitis cases[35] here in three weeks than during my whole training. In our two tents of surgical patients of one line (16 patients in each), we have four very ill peritonitis cases & one convalescent, also a bad typhoid perforation. But they are splendid patients & do wonderfully well in spite of the flies, & a certain amount of infection due to excessive perspiration.

Have I mentioned our latest comfort is a bath room – a small enclosure, with cement floor, & galvanized iron roof & walls, with the bath in the centre, with a limited supply of water? A large watering cart is filled just outside, & a pipe attached, so all we have to do is to turn on the tap. Of course as there are 29 of us to use the same tub, it cannot be a daily luxury, but it's simply great to get one occasionally.

...

...[O]ur Matron has gone to England on sick leave for a month or six weeks, leaving a Miss Hunter[36] in charge, a sister who has been her assistant for months, a pretty attractive girl with a great deal of tact, & so a good one to have in the office.

We are hoping daily for re-inforcements, but so far no word of them. [N]o one seems to know [w]hether they have been asked for, but certainly they are badly needed. Only two Sisters are off duty at present, one with a broken clavicle (fell over a tent-rope on night-duty), the other with a nasty attack of jaundice. [T]hen one is the Acting Matron, three on night-duty, two in the Operating Room, leaving 21 on day duty to look after just over 400 patients, the majority of whom need a great deal of nursing. Of course we can only do our best & let the rest go; one simply wouldn't last out a month [without] some time off duty every day.

We hear two more hospitals have just arrived & are to be stationed near here. [W]hether this means a move for some who have been here a long time, or whether it is by way of preparation, no one seems to know – or perhaps I should say no one has told us.

...

Ever yours lovingly
　　Lollie.

Temp. now 101 – still going up. Have I ever asked you to make me an odd veil & plain slip-waist in your spare moments? Mildred & I are both [in] need, & haven't the energy to commence & make them.

Letter No. 73
Salonika
July 10th, 1916

Dear Mother,

Very many happy returns of a month from to-day.... Yesterday I sent you off a cable to let you know the Organ had at last put in an appearance, & is a tremendous success. Although we have a fairly decent piano in the Sisters' Anteroom, it cannot be used for the church services, as the tent where they are held is a long distance from our lines. [C]onsequently we continue to use the little tin-pan affair given us when on Lemnos, since when each week the tone seems to have become smaller & more squeaky.... Really the organ is a little beauty, & everyone is simply delighted with it, especially our Padre.

The same day the organ arrived, several of the boxes sent off sometime in December & January turned up – of course the excitement!!! But you can imagine our disgust on opening them to find they had all been opened & gone over, apparently in England, [&] very badly re-packed, the box containing my Xmas Cake in particularly bad condition. Doesn't it seem too bad?

Of the base-ball outfit, only the mitt was left, & no note, so haven't the donator's name in order to acknowledge it. By the way, don't let on to her some of it was lost – it's too disappointing – & the men were delighted to get even the mitt....

Now that Mildred & I are on the lines again, we are simply delighted to have these extras, & those nice pyjamas & extra towels are a god-send. There is so much malaria, patients running Temps of 104 & 105, who need to be changed constantly, & it's such a relief to have a private stock to draw on when the others run out. Really *everything* that we got is most useful, & *all* the articles treasures in themselves.

We haven't been able for some time to buy any baking powder, so the Mess Sister was greatly relieved when I handed her over what you had sent....

I feel very proud of myself to think I am so well, & mighty thankful, for even the men who have spent years in India say they "can't stick it here" – that is their favorite expression. I imagine it is the humidity they find so trying; of course being so close to the sea, it can't be a very dry climate. It's wonderful how the sun shines day after day – not a cloud – nor a drop of rain!
...

Well dear I must ... say good-bye to you for the present. This was really supposed to have been a birthday letter, but have mentioned little beyond the heat & the boxes. Of course I think it's wonderful what you have managed to do in the latter line, but if only you were here to fully realize what a help every single article has been, you would, I am sure, more than feel repaid.

... [E]very good wish in the world for the coming year,

> As ever Yours lovingly
> Lollie.

Letter No. 74
Salonika
July 20th, 1916

Dear Mother,

The past two days have been wonderfully cool – the first time in seven weeks that the thermometer has remained below the 100 mark in the shade for 24 hours – you can imagine the relief! I intended to have answered several letters that I owe, but we have been having such huge doses of quinine that I'm practically good for nothing beyond absolutely necessary work. Drugs certainly don't agree with me, but of course it's necessary, for there is a great deal of malaria around. Fortunately it is not serious, but the after effects are so disagreeable that I'd just as soon escape it, & apparently faithful quinine takers usually do.

...

Yesterday I set to work & fixed up our service tent, using the last of the chintz you sent to cover the linen cup-board. It has been splendid, & the hammer & tacks almost a daily joy.

...

Had a line from Temple saying he was now in the Royal Flying Corps & having a wonderful time. Poor Uncle will worry himself to death. I do feel sorry for him, & yet can quite understand Temple's feelings. Of course once the war is over, it's the best place in the world for him & will probably be an incentive to use what brains he has, whereas the Army Service Corps or military life in any other form would develop him socially ... but certainly not mentally.

Well dear I've no thoughts of any kind but wanted you to know Mildred & I are O.K. It's too hot to say more for the present....

As ever
Lollie.

Salonika
August 6th, 1916

My dear Cairine,

...

Was so glad to get your letter from St. Andrews dated 18th of June. By the time this reaches you, you will be back in Rockland enjoying the tomatoes & corn!

... Five more of our sisters were invalided to England a couple of days ago, & as six went in June, it made us pretty short. To our delight six arrived yesterday, so it helps us out. We are very busy, chiefly with Malaria. It is very prevalent here, & we are all taking quinine steadily.

Of course when I tell you I am once more on the casualty list, you will wonder if I am ever off! It is boils this time!![37] I got a nasty one on my right arm, but managed to keep on duty. I had it opened & my arm was very painful. The next horror was to find one coming near my right eye on the cheek bone. I was then forced to go off duty & apply fomentations for 24 hours. My face got swollen beyond recognition & my eye disappeared altogether. Next thing was to have an anaesthetic & have it lanced. Of course, as usual, I was deathly sick after the performance. It is getting on well & today I have the packing out & the swelling is going down, but I fear I shall always have a scar as a souvenir of Salonika! The enforced stay in bed has not been unwelcome, for I was tired & my head troubled me with all the inflammation.

We have had it very warm, but today the temp has dropped 30°, so of course we are nearly shivering.

...

August 7th

Strangely enough we had a regular downpour of rain all night, which will lay the dust & help generally. It is cool & damp today & it makes one realize how much we are going to suffer with cold. We will endure agony with Canadian winters "after the war."

We are all getting sick of roughing it – not that we are not a thousand times more comfortable than in Lemnos – but the thought of a comfortable house & a few luxuries appeals strongly.

Last week we had an interesting time in Salonika. Our ambulance was broken down, but Lollie & I thought we would take our chance on getting a lift. So we started forth on the dusty road, but soon hailed a lorry which took us a short distance, then some officers picked us up in their Ford – so we felt quite stylish! We spent quite a time poking about the Jewish & Turkish quarters. They all live in the most primitive fashion. [T]he shops, which are like shop windows on the street, are most interesting. Only one type of article [is] sold in each shop.

Then the brass & copper workers were most fascinating to watch. In another place about 6x10 feet in size, they were making old fashioned steelyards,[38] every bit made by hand. There were four men making the various [parts] – they had a forge – the bellows looked big enough for ten! The finished article stands about four feet, & I am sure was used in the dark ages.

In spite of all the interesting things we see, I should never advise anyone to come to Salonika on a pleasure trip!

...

Excuse the scrawl written in bed, & with much love to you all.

Affect. yours.
  Mildred.

Letter No. 77
S.S. Braemar Castle
August 17th, 1916

Dear Mother,

... [B]y the time these few lines reach Montreal, you will have heard by cable from London of our arrival there, & so the above address will not be any surprise.

The first we knew of this un-expected change was on Sunday night [Aug 13th], when at dinner the Acting Matron handed Mildred a cable from London, saying we (Mildred & self) were to be prepared to leave for England on 48 hours' notice. Nothing can give you any idea of the shock ... of disappointment the news gave us both, for there is every possibility ... of ... something doing in these parts shortly, & [we] would like to be in the midst of it. [T]hen of course we know & like the girls here & rather dread the thought of starting out afresh with a new unit. However, an order is an order, & it's not worthwhile kicking, for in the end we might lose by it, & at least we are being re-called to-gether & so feel we have no right to grumble.... [C]ertainly the change will do Mildred good, for she is looking miserable, & having all these boils has taken a lot out of her.

Needless to say we are most curious to know just why we are being re-called.... The majority are inclined to think that Mildred will have a position offered her as Matron. What we are inclined to think [is that] our Matron, who is in England, is having things her own way, which is to have the old girls re-called one by one & gradually have a fresh lot that she hopes to manage a little more easily than she has been able to manage us. And thirdly, it is just possible that many Sisters with influence are clamouring for foreign service, & so the Matron-in-Chief is recalling gradually those who have done a year's service, & so giv[ing] them a chance. Time will tell, & meanwhile, I ... am not going to worry but intend to enjoy the trip to England as much as possible. Of course it is not the pleasantest time of the year for these waters, but we don't feel the heat as much as we did this time last year....

... After this news, we did nothing but talk *all* evening [&] saw the O.C. ... [On] Tuesday during my hours [off], did as much packing as possible, &

in the middle of it, a box arrived for Mildred & another for myself, so had to unpack these & distribute the contents as we thought best. Really they were lovely boxes, & I couldn't help but feel disappointed that I wouldn't have the pleasure of distributing their contents to the patients....

You can well imagine I went to bed dead tired, for the work on the Lines has been very heavy recently, & knowing there was a good holiday ahead of me, felt it was up to me to do my share of the work as long as possible....

That evening Miss Scoble gave a little farewell party for us in her hut, inviting just a few of the old girls. It was quite an elaborate one, & she had spent her afternoon off duty in Salonica shopping for the event. Imagine having Coffee & liqueurs, followed by Musk Melon ... & delicious ice-cream & fancy cakes – & a large assortment of cigarettes! The organ arrived with the guests, so we had various songs, ending up with mournful hymns!!! Just why the latter it is difficult to say, except that they sound better than anything else....

Well the next morning, I was awakened at four o'clock to find Mildred having the most awful cramps followed by the Lemnos trouble.[39] I spent the whole morning finishing packing, a most disheartening job, for there is of necessity so much to be given & thrown away, & it is rather worrying to know just what to keep. One naturally collects so much, but it is impossible to pack it all....

... [W]e left the Hospital at 4.30 p.m. (August 16th), an ambulance being sent for us, & ... the Acting Matron & two of our Officers came down to see us off, & were allowed to come out on the tender & have dinner with us on the Braemar Castle. Unfortunately I developed one of my real bad headaches & was forced to go immediately to bed dinner-less, but feel quite O.K. to-day. The whole atmosphere of the boat is particularly nice. There are not very many patients, the Matron most pleasant & anxious that we should be as comfortable as possible, & the O.C. evidently not at all the interfering kind. We did not get up for breakfast, but our cabin got so warm about 11 a.m. we were forced to dress & go on deck where we have remained ever since....

The boat just glides along, for there is scarcely a ripple on the sea, which each hour becomes a more intense blue. On our way out we scarcely ever came close to shore ... but to-day we have passed quite close to several islands, which look most interesting, with here & there a small village built entirely of a pure white stone, right on the side of a hill.

Then a short time ago we passed a school of what appeared to be sponges, or whatever they are called when alive. You can't imagine how peaceful & quiet it seems away from the whole unit. Although surrounded ... by people, it is not so necessary to converse with strangers, & when you do it is not the same. Although we both feel rather tired out we are enjoying to the full being off alone once more.

...

August 19th, 1916. Saturday.

Yesterday was warm & muggy, but turned cooler in the afternoon & was quite comfortable on deck, but very warm in our stateroom. To-day is not so bad as there is a breeze blowing, but of course it is scarcely an enjoyable time of year for the Mediterranean.

Last night we went a good deal out of the regular course as we received an S.O.S. wire, but so far have seen nothing.

Poor Mildred has another boil on her jaw, [&] consequently [is] feeling quite miserable. I do hope as we strike a cooler clime the miserable things will disappear for good. Perhaps after all being re-called is the best thing that could have happened [to] us both. Anyway it is always a satisfaction to feel that whatever happens one didn't kick, but did as we were told.

...

August 26th, 1916

A great many days seem to have elapsed since I commenced this epistle, but there was no object in posting a letter in Malta, as we will probably be in England just as soon as any mail steamer.

Well I must go back a little. We arrived at Malta about 2 p.m. August 20th but it was 6 p.m. before we dis-embarked, when we were sent to a convalescent home for Nursing Sisters in an ambulance. Our hearts rather sank when we saw the place, a barren rambling house, where we received no welcome but were left to shift for ourselves. The sleeping apartment was rather like a ward, a large room containing about seven beds & absolutely no comforts, not even enough chairs to go round, not a nail to hang one's clothes on, one dim gas jet, & a general air of discomfort. Meals poor & scanty, but in spite of it all we got rather to like the place & would like to have remained longer than we were allowed.

... The next morning we went to town with some of the Sisters who knew the ropes, & found we had quite a distance to go to the shopping centre, as we were in a suburb called Sliema. [T]ook the ferry to Valletta & then a carrozza[40] to the Main Street & just wandered around until lunch, after which we had a rest & returned to town about 4 p.m. & had a good look at

St. Johns Cathedral, but Mildred was feeling so miserable we didn't attempt much. The following day she had a temperature & so stayed in bed in the morning, but at noon, hearing we were to depart in the early morning for England, I hustled into town to do a little shopping for us both & see what I could. Poor girl, she felt too miserable even to attempt it.

To me, even at this wrong season of the year, Malta is simply fascinating, & certainly if ever I have the opportunity, shall try & come back again. It has much of the charm of the East, with but few of its drawbacks. I found the glare very trying, for it is built entirely of white sand stone, & at this season of the year the sun is so intense, it is most trying. But the whole place is so quaint, the streets so immaculate, the people so polite & attentive, & the view at every turn glorious....

The Carrozza are the quaintest old things, covered over more or less like a four poster bedstead. The curtains are of linen & always seem clean. But they are not exactly luxurious for they have no springs. [H]owever as the charge is sixpence a mile, one can't complain.

...

The following morning (August 23) went on board the Braemar Castle again, much to our delight, & we sailed about noon. Poor Mildred had a chill about 4 p.m., her Temp. went up to 104-⅘ [F, 40.4 °C], & so un-doubtably had Malaria – must have got the bug just before leaving. It has made us realize how wise we were not to have objected to leaving, for she would have been invalided almost immediately, & in all probability I would have been left behind. But hasn't she been un-fortunate, & to-day she had to have another small boil opened on her right arm. She really is looking miserable & will have to have a rest.

The O.C. of this boat has also given me a letter to the Matron-in-Chief saying I am very anemic & suffering from debility & should have a rest. I really am feeling pretty fair but two or three weeks rest won't do me any harm.

Since we passed Gibraltar ... it has been frightfully rough, un-usually so even for the Bay of Biscay, & in spite of Mothersills, I had a pretty bad time – I still feel none too good. We expect to land in the morning, probably at Southampton, & will go direct to London, when I will cable you. Thought it foolish to send word from Salonica for knew you would worry all the time we were on the water....

...

As ever, Yours lovingly
Lollie.

August 31st, 1916

P.S. Arrived Southampton 8 a.m. Disembarked at noon. Had lunch in town & took 2.48 train to London. Will post this on arriving.

Always love from Lollie.

Sent Cable from Southampton.

5

England:
Officers and Honours

L aura and Mildred arrived in London just in time to experience the largest Zeppelin air raid of the war on the night of September 2, 1916. The noise from the bombs and the anti-aircraft guns was enough to make them leap out of bed, groping for their clothing. An attack from the air, Laura wrote to her mother, "is always more or less un-consciously on our minds," because they had undergone several raids in Salonika. At that point, Laura had mentioned only two of these raids to her mother, leavening the danger with humour, a strategy she followed whenever danger seemed to threaten. London would suffer additional raids, but tellingly, neither Laura nor Mildred mentioned them. More than 500 civilians were killed and more than 1,300 injured in air raids in England during the war.[1]

Matron-in-Chief Macdonald had recalled the two because she wanted Mildred as her assistant through "a time of bitter controversy" for the CAMC. On July 31, 1916, Colonel Herbert A. Bruce was appointed special inspector general to look into the organization and administration of the CAMC; he then replaced Major General G.C. Jones as administrative head for a short time; Jones was reappointed, but a major shakeup of personnel took place.[2] One of the main issues was whether to segregate Canadian soldiers in Canadian hospitals; underlying this dispute was Canadian nationalism and identity. Laura, despite her dislike of British authority, was in favour of continuing to cooperate with the British.

Given the controversy, Macdonald's choice of Mildred to replace her current assistant showed much trust in Mildred's abilities and discretion. And perhaps Mildred's influential family connections might be useful if changes threatened the administration of nurses. Certainly, Mildred's connections and administrative abilities made her, to Miss Macdonald, representative of the best of Canadian society and of the CAMC nursing cohort. Macdonald's patronage benefited both Laura and Mildred: not only had she brought them both to England, signalling her approval of their friendship, but she had also made them members of her club, invited them to dinner in her home, offered them tickets to special events, and taken a (sometimes reluctant) Mildred for drives and for tea with the Astors.

Laura was stationed at No. 1 Hyde Park Place, a Canadian hospital for officers in London. The luxurious Christmas of 1916 at this hospital contrasts sharply with the impoverished Christmas on Lemnos, where Mildred had improvised decorations with cotton stuck on paper with vaseline. This indulgent day for patients ended with privilege for Mildred and Laura: they were invited for Christmas dinner with Macdonald, giving us a rare glimpse of the matron-in-chief's private life.

Unusually, and with the matron-in-chief's approval, Laura was allowed to room with Mildred in a private hotel in London instead of living in residence in the hospital. Freed from hospital restrictions, the two revelled in being back "in civilization," indulging in theatres, concerts, leaves in cathedral towns, and dinners with returned colleagues from CSH No. 1. In spite of this patronage, Laura remained suspicious of the matron-in-chief's motives – an underlying theme that undercut her delight at being awarded the Royal Red Cross.

Macdonald indulged the friendship even further by arranging for Mildred to have leaves and free time when Laura did.[3] One such leave tested Laura's loyalties: just as she and Mildred were about to journey to Devon for a much-needed rest, Laura received word that her cousin Temple, a pilot, had crashed over enemy lines. His fate would remain unknown for several weeks. Laura was torn between staying in London to try to find out more about Temple from the War Office and taking Mildred, still suffering from the malaria she had caught in the east, on vacation. Laura's immediate concern for her friend won out, demonstrating the strength of their bond.

But despite their enjoyment of London, the two chafed at being in England when their professional skills were needed on active service and looked forward eagerly to Mildred's release from the office and to Macdonald fulfilling her promise to send them to France. Their time in Salonika and their medical leave in England meant they had missed the major battles fought in 1916 on the Western Front, including Verdun and the Battle of the Somme. But in the spring of 1917, the Battle of Arras and the Canadian success at Vimy Ridge gave urgency to their repeated requests for active service, as wounded Canadian officers filled Laura's hospital, Hyde Park Place.

Letter No. 77 & 78
London
September 3rd, 1916

Dear Mother,

The bomb has fallen & we now know why we were re-called! The Matron-in-Chief has to increase her office staff, & wants Mildred for the job, which of course means we will have to be separated. So far there is no news as to where I am to land, but no doubt it will be in England, & probably near London. Of course we are both disappointed, for we had hoped to remain to-gether – however we can't altogether pick & choose, & after all it is an honor for Mildred.

Once having laid eyes on us, Miss Macdonald realized we both needed a holiday, especially Mildred, so we were both "boarded" & given five weeks leave. I think had we pressed the point very hard we might have been able to get leave to Canada, but it would have meant coming up before a special board ... & longer leave, & as Miss M. is more or less waiting for Mildred, it hardly seemed fair. And much as I would love to see you, I dread the trip to & fro, for it would mean 20 days on the sea & about the same on land, & after our experience in the Bay of Biscay, I feel the trip would do me little good, whereas five weeks spent quietly here ought to put me on my feet again.

Now that we are away from the unit & routine, we realize how tired we are, & Mildred is decidedly "nervy." She says the traffic in London nearly sends her crazy.

... [On] Sept. 1st we reported at 86 The Strand,[4] where after the usual wait, we came up before the board, & both were given our leave. The joke is I got six weeks & Mildred only five, in spite of her really needing it more than I do, but of course if she is not well at the end of that time, they will prolong her leave.[5]

It seems Miss Macdonald now likes all the Sisters when not on duty to wear mufti,[6] so on leaving the office, we started on a round of shopping. Our whole out-fit is in a terrible state ... mufti was our first consideration after ... visiting the bank.[7]

...

At 2 a.m. we were awakened by the air-raid.[8] I think since being in Salonica, it is always more or less un-consciously on our minds, for the first shot always has me right out of bed, looking for bed-room slippers.... For some reason or another, it is less up-setting here than when more in the open, although I imagine the London raids are far more dangerous. However in any case one's chance of being hurt is of course very small.

This morning we awoke to find it raining again. I really don't mind it, in fact find it rather a relief after the eternal sun-shine of the East, but wish I were a little better prepared for it. My raincoat won't be here until to-morrow. ...

Of course I am just longing to hear from you after you have heard of the move. The one reason I am really pleased is that I know you will be relieved. ...

   Always love dear. Will write in a few days again.
      Ever yours lovingly
         Lollie.

Laura and Mildred toured the Lake District in England, then went on a brief trip around Scotland. They luxuriated in the "freshest of boiled eggs, thin bread & butter, and the richest of coffee" for their breakfasts, and revelled in the peace and quiet of country walks, the architecture and shops of Edinburgh, and tours of castles and cathedrals. After the tribulations of hospitals in the East, it was a well-deserved time of recuperation.

                                                       Letter No. 83
                                                             London
                                               October 4th, 1916

Dear Mother,

   Well our travelling days for a little time are over, [&] although I don't actually start in to work again for another week, have quite a busy time ahead of me....
...

   ... I went with Mildred, who had to report, & fortunately we both had a good talk with Miss Boulter, now a Matron & Miss Macdonald's assistant. Miss M. is a Major you know!! Mildred ... goes to the office on Friday, & I don't go to work until the following Friday, when I am to be in the Daughters of the Empire Hospital for Officers only, No. 1 Hyde Park Place.

When we first arrived, Miss Boulter had promised Mildred we would be able to room together – now it seems if we do so it will be at my own expense.[9] We have talked it over & if we can get a room anywhere in the vicinity, have decided to do so for a time at least.... Mildred dreads rooming alone, for her work will be rather up-hill for a time, & living alone in London is desperate; we would see but little of one another otherwise, as her time off duty will rarely be the same as mine, & now that the place is so dark after daylight has gone, one can't go out much at night with any degree of comfort. She wants to pay for me, but don't think I will let her, for of course I shall be much more comfortable living like that than I would be in the crowded quarters I would otherwise have. Don't read this part out to *anyone* except Uncle....

Always love dear from Lollie.

Letter No. 84
19 Portman St.,
Portman Square
London
October 10th, 1916

Dear Mother,

...

Our room, while not very large, seems palatial after our old canvas hut, & now that we have un-packed ... & got rid of our camping outfit ... looks quite comfortable & roomy.... On the ground floor there is a lounge where we can smoke, & where after-dinner coffee is served. On the floor above there is a very comfortable drawing-room, furnished in good taste, nice mahogany, & large easy chairs ... the latter covered in good-looking chintz. This house was taken over for a private Hotel only this spring, consequently all wall papers are fresh, white paint throughout, & all new bed-room furniture, giving the whole place a fresh clean look. Of course being able to have her meals on the spot makes all the difference to Mildred, & as prices have gone up everywhere, do not think she is paying too much. Anyway we could find nothing cheaper. I am barely five minutes' walk from my hospital, two minutes from the Tube, half a minute from Oxford Street, & five minutes from Selfridges, so you see we are in a splendid position. As I will probably have to be at the hospital early, felt I must be close. Mildred does not go to the office until 9.30 so it doesn't matter so much to her.

...

The following morning[10] Mildred reported for duty, & I collected our belongings & moved, a whole morning's job. Mildred came up to our new abode for lunch, [& we] flew for the remainder of the afternoon, in fact until nine. We un-packed after lunch, then wandered out to get one or two necessary odds & ends, & arrived back to find a note from Temple.... I can't tell you ... how delighted I was to see him, & it has made me realize that I am just as fond of him as of our own boys. Of course he is very boyish & casual but I do think he was genuinely glad to see me.... He always was good-looking but is especially attractive at present, & seems so happy & contented. I was pleased though to hear him say he was most anxious to finish his college course once the war was over. I do hope he sticks to that....

...

    Heaps of love always
      from Lollie.

Letter No. 85
London
October 16th, 1916

Dear Mother,

...

... [O]n Saturday I went to my new job, & certainly everyone has been very nice. There are eight Sisters & 26 patients, so if they leave the whole of the present staff, ought to have a fairly easy time this winter.[11] Of course I don't care for this type of nursing (Officers!) but one can't have everything, & I feel rather pleased to have a little easier time than we had all the time we were in the East. Of course until one gets on to the place & their way of doing things, it is rather worrying – but a week or two will get one over that. And even if we get very busy, it is nice to start in when the work is not heavy. The place is full, but a great many of the patients are up & around, & so beyond perhaps helping them – seeing to their meals, & doing a few dress-ings – there is little else, giving us plenty of time to look after the really sick ones. Several leave this week, so will probably get sick ones in their place. In the meantime it's mighty nice, & as I say, the girls seem a decent lot.

There are rumours going the round that the General in charge of Medical Affairs (I won't mention names) is in dis-favor with S[am] H[ughes] & that there may be a tremendous change soon all round. Certainly if the segregat-ing of the Canadian Hospitals is what S.H. wants, I think the latter is the one to be put out. To me it seems a tremendous mistake, & will do away or

rather cause a great deal of ill-feeling between the C.A.M.C & the R.A.M.C.
Undoubtably there are a great many things in favor of it, but far more
against. I wonder what the people at home think. I only hope the Lady
Drummond type[12] are strong enough to have some say....

...

>   Lovingly
>   Lollie.

*Laura's Uncle George Hadrill came to London to visit his son, Temple, about to
leave for France, for several weeks in late November and early December. Laura
was on night duty and had a severe cold during his visit, so her uncle took Mildred
to dinner and the theatre instead, treating her like a family member. Throughout
the fall and winter, Laura also recounted meetings with Helen Fowlds, a member
of CSH No. 1 who had returned from Salonika, and a number of other nurses
from their former unit.*

>   Letter No. 97
>   No. 1 Hyde Park Place
>   London W.
>   December 25th, 1916[13]

Dear Mother,

    Xmas is over & altogether we had a very happy day, though the night
following was somewhat of a nightmare, for I never was so sleepy in my life!!
However was in bed in good time this morning & had the best sleep I have
had since I went on night duty.
    ... Nothing of interest happened Xmas Eve. We hung up stockings for all
the patients, which they thoroughly appreciated, & earlier in the evening
decorated the Xmas tree, which was in the big Ward, all the bed patients
having been moved down from the up stair[s] wards until the festive season
is over. The stockings came from Toronto, net affairs filled with the usual
mixture of sweets, nuts, cigs, tobacco, playing cards, etc. The girls during the
day had decorated the ward & halls. We had practically no evergreen – it
was so expensive – but an abundance of holly, mistletoe, & laurel, so [were]
able to make the place look very Xmasy. Of course the holly here is lovely,
the leaves so bright & fresh looking. As we have only one really sick patient,
Miss Thompson & I managed to get a good rest & so prepare for what
promised to be a strenuous day.

... [On Xmas Day] I met Mildred (did I mention she had gone down to Cheyne Place with Miss Macdonald for the week end?) at our own Hotel & we went around the corner to the Church of the Annunciation, where we had a nice but very high service ... at 9.30 a.m. One felt it was all most reverent, but deep down in my heart, I prefer a simple service. From there we went home, opened up our mail, & it was twelve before I got to bed. Mildred gave me two very dainty night gowns, two books, & a few choice cigarettes – altogether she was most extravagant. I got up at 3.30, dressed in uniform, & went over to our Xmas tree. Mrs Gooderham, General Jones & his wife & a host of others were there,[14] & everyone entered into the spirit of the thing & thoroughly enjoyed themselves. There was a nice little present for each patient, Sister, Orderly & maid from the I.O.D.E. in Toronto.... Then the patients had clubbed to-gether & presented each Sister with three pairs gloves, the package being attached to a funny doll of some description with a piece of poetry.... My rag doll was an awful looking soldier dressed in khaki, with bulgy knees, & flat feet, & flapping ears!

Tea was served those who could [go] to the dining-room, which looked very pretty. Many of the old patients had sent in flowers, which helped a lot to brighten up the rooms. At first I had intended to have dinner here, but when I found, owing to there being so many convalescent patients, I could stay off late ... decided to have dinner with Mildred at Cheyne Place, Miss Macdonald having invited me.... This is ... the first time I have really had anything to say to Miss Macdonald, & ... was rather glad of the opportunity of meeting her. She is a fearfully erratic woman, clever, & certainly wonderfully good company.... [T]he dinner ... was plain but very nice – grape fruit, turkey, vegetables, chestnut dressing, plum pudding, nuts, raisins, cocktails, & champagne. Played bridge for a while & I left about 11.15 p.m. so as to make sure of a bus.... Then came the trying time – I was so sleepy I positively felt sick. However got through the night & to-day had a fine sleep, & certainly Xmas was a great success altogether, though the only absolutely satisfactory place to spend it is at home. [But] the patients appreciated what we did, so it made it worthwhile. They had quite a gay dinner here, [the] up-patients having it with the Sisters who were in, & all having champagne & port, & everyone went to bed with a whiskey & soda.

...

Heaps of love dear always & best wishes for the New Year from Lollie.

London
February 24th, 1917

Dear Mother,

Mildred tells me she has sent you a cable this morning to let you know I had received the Royal Red Cross!! Don't be too puffed up about it, for it's more or less luck as to *who* gets it, & there are many who should have it in No. 1 Stationary if I should.

The pleasure has been rather spoilt by Mildred not receiving hers at the same time, for I know she was recommended ahead of me – but for reasons un-known she didn't. I imagine someone thought it wiser to wait until she was out of the Office, for I feel sure she will have one in the end. Of course the nicest part of it all is I shall probably have a glimpse inside Buckingham Palace.

A great many of [the] No. 1 girls have got it, but I feel awfully badly [that] one or two who worked if anything harder & more cheerfully than most of us, haven't. That's the fly in the ointment. However I take what the Gods send & am thankful even if I don't deserve it.

Please don't say much about it & this note is just between ourselves. Mildred of course is making the most of the opportunity to shower me with attentions. She more than spoils me.

Forgive haste but wanted to write immediately. Always love from L.

Letter No. 110
London
March 2nd, 1917

Dear Mother,

...

Many thanks to you & Uncle George for the cable congratulating me. The great day is to be to-morrow & we go to Buckingham Palace to be invested, & I believe afterward to meet Queen Alexandra.... Did I mention that Boultbee, Acting Matron during Miss Tremayne's absence in Canada, & Sister Rose at No. 1 Hyde Park Place also received the R.R.C.? [B]oth awfully nice girls & splendid workers from Vancouver. Of course we all go together, which makes it very nice, but I am bitterly disappointed Mildred is not going with me, particularly knowing that she is bound to get it in the future, for she is more entitled to it than I am, but for some curious reason

Miss M. evidently thinks it wiser for her to receive it after leaving the Office. But I know her family, not understanding the circumstances, will wonder, & deep in her heart, I know Mildred feels it. Not that she grudges it to me for a minute – but just that we aren't going together.

Miss Macdonald offered her the Matronship of a large hospital just being opened in England, but Mildred has refused it & asked to be left just a Nursing Sister. I can't quite make up my mind whether she is wise to do so or not. It would mean a great deal of worry for the first few months & probably that she would remain in England [for] the duration of the war, & while she doesn't want to be separated from me, I am sure Miss Macdonald would leave us to-gether. [B]ut you know it would be difficult for us to have our time off to-gether, & it isn't altogether wise for a Matron to have a special friend in the Unit, unless as her assistant, which would mean we could never be away to-gether at any time.[15]

At any rate, she has definitely turned it down, so don't know just what will happen next. If you run into any of her relatives, just drop a hint you heard she had been offered the position but refused it, for I know she never will....
...

Our little dinner on Monday night [given by the nurses at No. 1 Hyde Park Place to honour the R.R.C. nurses] was just amongst ourselves, Mildred being the only invited guest. We had our usual mess meal with a few additions, such as commencing with grape-fruit, [&] ending with the most delicious ice-cream & chocolate sauce, also candies, salted almonds, sparkling Moselle, & liqueur. It really was awfully nice of them.

Thursday (yesterday) as Miss Macdonald had invited Mildred & I to dine with her, I asked for last hours.

Did I ever mention that Miss M. was now living in rather a nice bachelor apartment in St. James Court? I'm not quite sure how she got hold of it, but the owner put it at the disposal of someone doing war work & she was lucky enough to get it. A large living room, plainly but beautifully furnished, the owner evidently a great lover of Japanese or Chinese art, for there were several beautiful prints, the only other pictures being an oil-painting over the mantle & an exquisite water-color.

Then there's a comfortable bed-room & a lovely bath-room. We had dinner in the living-room. You can either have your meals served in your own room or go to the restaurant. I was so glad she decided on the former. We didn't commence dinner until after 8 o'clock, & Miss M. was in a very talkative mood. When finally we said we must go, we nearly fainted when we found it was 12.45!! No taxi was to be had, & so there was nothing for us but to walk home. It was a gorgeous night & [we] really rather enjoyed it, but it made it quite late getting home. Fortunately to-day I had the whole day off, & so was able to sleep in, although poor Mildred had to get up....

Well I think I have brought you pretty well up to date, & will send you a line probably on Sunday telling you of my meeting with "George." Of course I am keenly interested in seeing Buckingham Palace ... but rather dread the ordeal. Fortunately have a new cotton uniform coming home to-night, which is lucky as my old ones are very shabby, & we have to appear in our working uniform.... Heaps of love dear always

from Lollie.

[P.S.] ...

Letter No. III
London
March 4th, 1917

Dear Mother,

Well the great day is over, & like most affairs one dreads, the ordeal wasn't so bad as we had anticipated. Of course it was all intensely interesting, even to get one's nose inside the Palace, but I must begin from the beginning.

We received a telegram on Thursday night saying an investiture was to be held at Buckingham Palace at 10 a.m. Saturday, with orders to appear in service uniform.[16] Of course it made such a difference four of us going to-gether, Boultbee, Rose & Fowlds, the latter one of the old members of No. 1 Stationary who is now at Bushy Park. As we had to go in veils & only our little capes, needless to say had a taxi, which we had wait for us. Immediately on entering the Palace, several flunkies came forward to take our capes, etc., which were checked in a most business-like manner at a small stand in the hall apparently arranged for such occasions.

The footmen (or whatever one should call them) are dressed in black knickers & scarlet cut-away coats, but can't remember any details. I am not any too observant, my heart was more or less in my mouth at the thought of an abominable curtsey, & there was so much to see that a great many details escaped me. If only I had the opportunity again, am sure I could take in a whole lot more. By the way, these men had none of the severely grand manner one expected, but were more or less like human beings.

Having disposed of our capes, we were then ushered into a large room, entirely filled with small chairs, all neatly numbered, & we were then told in

what order we came, all being placed alphabetically, Imperial Sisters first &
Canadians afterward. We had quite a wait as the Officers receive their decorations first, but our signal came about 11.15.... [W]e all lined up, passing
through various rooms, where needless to say I kept my eyes open & took
in various things such as furniture, pictures, [&] china ... but as the line
kept moving steadily forward, couldn't loiter as much as I would have liked.
When we arrived at the room of rooms,[17] to my surprise, saw a line of
Indian Officers standing at attention, & what with gazing at them & then
collecting my thoughts enough to try & not disgrace my country, I didn't
notice anything else.

The King was most gracious – hung my medal on a hook which had
already been pinned on my uniform, shook hands & then asked what
Hospital I was working in. On hearing it was the I.O.D.E., he remarked,
"Oh! that is where Sister Tremaine is." Having been previously informed if
spoken to, to be sure & add Your Majesty the first time, & afterward Sir,
needless to say I forgot & used the latter! But really it wouldn't do to have
everything go correctly or poor George would have no fun at all, for I am
sure he gets a certain amount of amusement out of our mistakes. Knowing
I shall never speak to His Majesty again, I must give you the whole conversation. Then he said, "I hear she has gone to Canada, is it on a visit to her
family?" to which I replied "she had gone on transport duty, but hoped to
see her family when in Canada." It is just as well for him not to think we
run off & have too many holidays. With that he said, "Oh that will be very
nice for her" & so ended my one & only conversation with Royalty. I then
passed on, going out into the Hall, where my medal was taken from me,
placed in a box & returned. I waited until Sister Rose had gone through the
same performance, then with Fowlds & Boultbee we got into a taxi & went
over to *visit*! Queen Alexandra, having previously been requested by note to
do so. I really was awfully interested to see the interior of her home, but
frightfully disappointed when I saw it. The drawing-room we were in had ...
many beautiful things in it, but the whole place was so over-crowded [&]
the furnishings rather shabby – most un-attractive.

In a small room beyond we were presented to the Queen, but the place
was so small & the crowd so large that we were simply rushed through &
didn't get ... a chance to take in our surroundings at all. The Queen was
dressed in an old fashioned, very plain black tight tailor-made suit, a funny
little hat & heavy veil, so didn't look at all her best, but she was most gracious
as always, shook hands with each one of us, handing us afterward a book.
Some Red Cross book (I forget for the moment the exact title) & a small
picture, a nothing in itself, but interesting because of the giver....

... [18]

Certainly King George does everything in his power to make the men realize he appreciates what they are doing. Everybody seems to like him, & the men find him very easy to talk to & say there is very little formality at these affairs.

...

Bad news from France to-day – we haven't heard many details, but am afraid the Canadians have had a bad time of it.[19]

Always love to you
from Lollie.

P.S. Of course I'll never quite forgive Miss Macdonald for not giving Mildred the R.R.C. at the same time as I got it, [a]lthough I know she meant to do her a kindness – probably will end by giving her a 1st Class R.R.C. Mine is 2nd Class. I think all are except to Matrons.

Letter No. 116.
[April 1917]
London

Dear Mother,

...

We have had several men back from the Vimy Ridge encounter. They say it was wonderful, & everything went splendidly – no confusion, & the men went over smoking their pipes & cigarettes as though it were nothing un-usual. Of course the casualties are immense – but when one remembers the number of men there, 8,000 out of four divisions isn't such a big percent. But isn't it awful to think that may go on in-definitely....

My love to Uncle. I know how dreadfully he must be feeling these days. It is terrible for him.... Heaps of love dear always from Lollie.

In May 1917, Laura's cousin Temple was reported missing when his aeroplane crashed during a flight over the German lines. Laura and Mildred had been about to set off on leave when they received the news.

Letter No. 122
Paignton, Devon
May 20th, 1917

Dear Mother,

Of course I simply can't for a moment forget Uncle George, & much as I think of Temple & what he may be enduring as a prisoner in France, still he is young, & if alive one feels can stand the strain. [B]ut for Uncle it is too terrible for words – the awful suspense & un-certainty. Never have I felt so far from home as at present, & it seems such ages before I can have a line. Mr. Temple has made all possible enquiries & of course heard nothing further; I have written Miss Macdonald & through her feel I shall be able to get in touch more easily with the Casualty department than I could person-ally. [T]hen to-day I wrote the Squadron Command of the 54th, who I feel sure will tell me anything he can, & if it is different at all from Uncle's cable will cable it on. I hesitated about answering Uncle's cable for over a day, feeling it might be too great a disappointment receiving one that gave no news of Temple – then felt it would be such a long time before he could hear from me, decided to send it in your name, & so save him from any shock. Only hope it did not up-set you.[20]

And now for a confession. In writing Uncle George I really left him to understand the cable followed us here, because I was so afraid he would feel hurt that Mildred & I started off on a holiday under the circumstances, not realizing why it was necessary.

... [T]he cable did follow us, but just as the taxi was at the door & our luggage had been sent off, we got a phone message ... giving us the news & saying the cable would follow. The previous night, Mildred had had quite a bad attack of Malaria & was feeling very seedy.... I had to decide on the [spur of the] moment, & thought it better to go right on to Paignton ... especially as I realized we could do no real good in London. But I was so afraid Uncle might mis-understand that I didn't go into detail, but just told him the truth as far as it went ... & shall leave it to you to tell him what you think best.

Now that I am here, I really think it was the wisest thing to do, for I know from other people's experience how little one can find out personally at the War Office, & I feel sure Miss Macdonald will do all she can.

...

It's no good trying to realize it all for I can't! I wonder if it is something peculiar in myself, but to me it seems Temple must be alive as much as he ever was. But I cannot get Uncle out of my head. I can't tell you how glad I shall be to hear from you.

...

... Always love to you dear from Lollie.

Letter No. 123
Paignton, Devon
May 23rd, 1917

Dear Mother

... [T]he War Office have said they know nothing beyond the news they sent you. [S]till I have felt very much encouraged ... on hearing that the Germans so far have always reported any of the Flying Corps Officers killed in their country, although they never report either wounded or prisoners.... [W]hile it is terrible to think of Temple wounded & a prisoner.... I feel had he been killed, we surely would have heard by now. Then I have been told so often how much better the R.F.C. Prisoners have been treated than anyone else that there must be some truth in it....

...

It seems a long time since I have heard from you, & each day hope for a line. The thought of what you & Uncle have been going through this past week has made me think of so many things, & just how much you, Mother dear, mean to me. I suppose it is the Holland reserve that makes me say so little about it, but often since I have been away I have realized what a selfish daughter I have been to you at times, not through lack of love, but sheer thoughtlessness. The whole size of it is you have always been so un-selfish yourself, you have spoilt us all. Sometimes I wonder if this ... war will ever end, & life go on in the old way.

...

Did I mention I sent you a 2nd cable, thinking Uncle might be a little encouraged on hearing the Germans usually report all Officers killed in the R.F.C.? Doesn't it seem curious that they should treat the R.F.C. men with more consideration & respect than any others?

...

... Good night – my love to Uncle George. If only we could hear something definite what a comfort it would be – & yet I can't help but feel that no news means the best news in the end.

Ever so much love for your own self from Yours lovingly
Lollie.

Letter No. 126
Lyme Regis
June 1st, 1917

Dear Mother,

... [H]aving received this morning a most encouraging letter from Temple's O.C. in France, thought I would let you know at once. He tells me he has written Uncle also, & I hope that letter may have gone some time ago.... The gist ... was that other pilots in the same fight saw Temple's machine run along the ground for some distance, & on reaching some ploughed land, turned over. He goes on to say the machine they use always does so on ploughed land, & ... this is no cause for alarm as they frequently do the same on their own aerodrome, & at such a time it is practically impossible for the driver to be hurt. He adds that he feels almost sure Temple is un-hurt & only a prisoner, & I have since been thinking that perhaps he is safer as a prisoner than were he still at his work! Of course one does hear awful tales which un-doubtably are true of the treatment of prisoners in certain camps, but the R.F.C. men so far have been treated fairly well.... [Cousin] Nance[21] to-day was telling me of a friend of theirs, wounded some time ago & taken prisoner, who writes that he has met with nothing but kindness from his enemies. [S]o there is still hope, & even if in one of the bad camps, with his health & youth, one feels he will pull through alright. I feel ever so much more cheerful.

This morning's mail also brought me a letter from you, & I was so glad to get it.... I am so glad to hear that Uncle is standing the strain so well, & quite agree with you, it is far better for him to go to the office daily, for it will help him to pass the long hours of waiting.

...

... Always love to you from Lollie

Lyme Regis
June 1st, 1917

My dear Cairine,

...

We have been away on leave since May 17th. Just as we were starting, a cable came telling us Lollie's cousin, Temple Hadrill, who is in the Flying Corps, was Missing. She felt dreadfully, as they have been brought up together & the boy is more like a brother to her. We have made every in-quiry & today we received a note from the O.C. of the Squadron he was with saying he had great hopes of his being a Prisoner, so if so, we may hope he is still alive.

We went to Paignton, South Devon, which is a little place on the coast. Not the type of place I would enjoy to spend a holiday in, as it is too towni- fied. But as a centre it was simply splendid. We took some lovely walks, & I reduced my waist line considerably, (much to my delight!) for I had got very flabby sitting in that office all winter. We used to take our lunch with us & go for ... walks to various interesting little villages, ruined Castles, etc.

...

We managed a coaching trip to Dart Moor, but as the horses looked so thin, we felt rather ashamed to be pulled up so many hills – consequently we had to walk up a good many.

A couple of days ago we came on to Lyme Regis and are staying with relatives of Lollie's. They have a very comfortable old house, beautiful grounds & garden.... Tomorrow we return to London & report on June 4th.

Any minute after that we shall be shunted off to France, & I will be glad to be settled once more. Of course I rather dread the thought of a change – still one soon shakes down.

...

Our letters from France will be very heavily censored, so am afraid there will be little of interest that I can tell you. The Casualty Clearing Stations are quite far up the line – it is the nearest that women get to the front, without any danger of course to any of us.... I mean we are safe there, yet as close to things as women are allowed.[22] We get the men after they have passed through the Field Ambulances – we only keep them about 24 [to] 48 hours unless they are dangerously ill, then they are held over until it is safe to send them on to the Base Hospitals around Boulogne, Etaples or elsewhere. There are only about eight or ten nurses on the staff & they usually try & pick out fairly congenial people.

The best news we all could get would be to hear the war is over. Still until Germany is *well* beaten it cannot be considered.

... Affect. Yrs.
    Mildred.

Crowborough[23]
June 20th, 1917

My dear Cairine,

As we are not going to France for a month or so, I decided I had better make use of the money you sent. Upon consideration I decided to put £7-10- into the General Fund for Canadian Prisoners of War. The Canadian Red

Cross Society have a department especially for Canadian prisoners. I saw Jean Bovey at the office & told her where the money came from. She was very pleased to take the money, for she said they did not often get subscriptions for the *General* Fund, & there were so many prisoners without friends to look after them. She told me to tell you how pleased they were to get your subscription.

We are not going to France as soon as we had anticipated. I don't really mind as long as we get there before the cold weather sets in. The thought of another winter campaign is appalling. Yet I am sure we are in for a couple more at least.

At present we are at Crowborough, which is an ideal spot in the summer. We are on the direct line to Brighton, so the train service is good. The Hospital is ... a large house ... for Officers who are attached to the Canadian Camp here. We have no sick patients, & I say two house maids could do the work more efficiently than Lollie & I. However, we are enjoying it, for it is lovely country & we are never at a loss for something to do. The lack of work does not worry me, for there will be lots of that in France. (I mean work.)

My brother David's boy – Robin – is with the Canadian Engineers & is at present here in training. He is such a nice boy, just 17, & seems younger, though he has lots of common sense. He drops in & has dinner with us frequently, & is not at all upset at facing four elderly females. Last Sunday afternoon he was free so we decided to hire a "Ford" & take him to Eastbourne, a good excuse for an extravagance. Well, I felt well repaid, for certainly Robin enjoyed it. We had dinner there & got him home by ten p.m.

...

Our cottage we live in is very nice. Lollie & I have a nice bedroom with verandah. The house is a mass of roses. The flowers are wonderful here, & certainly Sussex is a lovely county.

I am wondering if you will be going to St. Andrews this year.

...

Hoping you are all well & with Much love to all –

Affectionately Yrs.
Mildred H. Forbes.

Letter No. 130
Crowborough, Sussex.
June 21st, 1917

Dear Mother,

... Mr. Temple wired me the good news; isn't it simply splendid? I never believed hearing anyone was a prisoner could cause so much joy, but it just goes to prove how one can change their minds on occasion; for really as no wound was mentioned in the wire, & after the C.O.'s letter, I think there is every chance of Temple having been taken prisoner un-hurt. You will have had ... my letter telling you I had made arrangements for a parcel to be sent, also cigarettes & bread, & have written Temple to let me know anything he wants. Karlsruhe un-doubtably is one of the most comfortable camps, & I have heard more liberty is granted there than most places. What a relief to Uncle to hear something definite – & really in my heart of hearts, now that we know the boy is alive, I think it is the very best thing that could have happened, for it is the _only_ chance a Pilot in a single-seated fighting machine has of being alive after the war. And while the boy may have hard-ships to contend with, the R.F.C. people have less than most from all ac-counts, & more liberty. It will be such a comfort to hear from the boy himself, though I realize ... he can say very little & nothing against the place. However he need say nothing un-true, & if he is allowed to play tennis & exercise ... & can write & obtain food & comforts, we will feel it might be worse.

Of course he is probably very disappointed at being out of it all – however he always has made the best of any unfortunate situation, & we can only hope & pray his cheerful disposition will help him over any hard road now.

...

My very best love to Uncle George always for Yourself.

Ever yours lovingly Lollie.

[P.S.] ...

Letter 133.
London
July 12th, 1917[24]

Dear Mother,

Our summons has come at last & we are now on our way to France....
Right after breakfast this morning had my hair waved, & then Mildred & I refused to go near a shop, & rushed down to have a look at Westminster Abbey.... Then we wandered through the cloisters & into the Close, & there

it was perfect & so peaceful!.... Then we took a bus to another restaurant on Old Compton St. & had another ... good lunch. Came up to Hotel, am writing to you, & leave at 5.20 for Folkestone. Imagine we will cross to-night, probably spend the night in Boulogne, & proceed to No. 2 Canadian Casualty Clearing in the morning....

Well I had better stop as time is going. We will have to be at [the] station a good ¾ hour ahead of time, in order to make sure of getting [our] luggage ... on in time. Travelling isn't what it used to be in peace times. Love to Uncle & heaps for Your self.

from Yours lovingly
Lollie.

6

France:
Trauma and Taking Charge

A published photograph of CCS No. 2 shows a reassuring permanency: the summer sun shines on well-kept buildings surrounded with flowers in bloom, two nurses relax on the island of grass beside the drive, and others bustle in and out of the buildings.[1] No wounded soldiers are in sight; they are hidden in the tents that fill the background. This peaceful picture would soothe any anxiety that relatives of nurses, medical staff, or patients might feel: a CCS, this photo tells us, is a tranquil place far from the battle area.

But CCS No. 2, where Mildred and Laura were posted in July 1917,[2] was neither peaceful nor safe. Located at Remy Siding, just south of Poperinghe in Belgium, it was a mere 15 kilometres from the Ypres salient, so subject to frequent air raids,[3] shelling, and threats of gas attacks. The two could see the flashes and feel the thunder of the guns at the front.

CCSs were the nearest that nurses could get to the trenches. Casualties walked or were carried by stretcher bearers to the nearest aid post or field ambulance to have first dressings done. They were then shipped by motor convoys and ambulance trains to the nearest group of casualty clearing stations for triage, treatment, and, if necessary, surgery. If possible, they were then evacuated down the line to the stationary and general hospitals or returned to their regiments. The clearing stations within a group, such as the Remy group, took turns receiving convoys so that no single CCS was overwhelmed. Bed capacity was between three hundred and six hundred. Patients seldom stayed more than forty-eight hours before being evacuated out, meaning that nurses did not get to know many of their patients or see their recovery.[4]

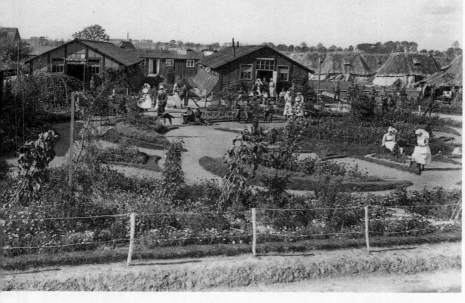

Casualty Clearing Station No. 2, Remy Siding, France. *George Metcalf Archival Collection, Canadian War Museum, CWM CCS219800795–003_2*

Mildred and Laura reported for duty at CCS No. 2 on July 14, 1917,[5] just in time to face the heavy bombardment of the German lines that preceded the Third Battle of Ypres (Passchendaele). On July 31 at 3:50 a.m., the Allies attacked in the Ypres sector across an 18 kilometre front, an offensive designed to remove the threat to the Channel ports and the need to maintain "the Ypres salient."[6] According to its war diary, the first thirty days of July, CCS No. 2 admitted 3,396 casualties; during the five days from July 31 to August 4, it admitted 3,566 casualties. On August 1, more than two thousand patients swamped the CCS, with convoys arriving by train at its front door, while other casualties arrived by motor at the back door; patients overflowed onto stretchers placed outside, in the rain. After this initial crisis, casualties continued to pour in from the fighting. The total number of admissions for August 1917 was 11,141, with 8,939 evacuations and 1,913 operations performed. For Laura and Mildred, it was a strenuous time: their patients on Lemnos and at Salonika had been mostly medical and lightly wounded, but now they were dealing with severely wounded and gassed soldiers. During crises, they would have worked flat-out with their colleagues, functioning on little sleep.

Mildred took over as acting matron on September 11, 1917, a weighty responsibility that she would carry for almost a year, with Laura at her side as a nursing sister. Acting Matron Forbes was officially responsible for the "general nursing arrangements of the hospital," ensuring the nurses performed their duties, maintaining discipline and "good conduct" among her nurses, and confirming the "cleanliness and good order" of the wards. She also trained orderlies and NCOs, administered supplies, wrote confidential reports about her nurses, and arranged for their leaves.[7] Unofficially, she was also responsible for maintaining the morale of the medical unit and the physical and mental welfare of her nurses, a charge that, in contrast to her reluctant participation in teas in Salonika, she undertook with zest and Laura's full support. Her administrative abilities were tested immediately when, in a single twenty-four-hour period in September,[8] CCS No. 2 admitted 1,326 casualties and performed 93 operations.[9] Renewed fighting in October[10] resulted in high casualties, with almost 9,000 admitted that month.[11] Fighting conditions throughout the Ypres Salient were appalling: the preliminary bombardment churned up the earth, while unexpected and continuous rain turned the battlegrounds to a thick, glutinous mud, "a hell on earth ... [that] has come to symbolize the whole of the war" for its horror.[12] The campaign finally ended when the Canadians and British captured Passchendaele on November 6.

Despite the dangers and the constant work, responsibility suited Mildred: after the first weeks, her letters radiate cheerfulness and confidence, as well as her determination to make her CCS the "best" in the army. Finally in charge herself, her abilities recognized and commended, she felt free to comment on the male medical staff and on her nurses. From September 1917 to August 1918, the period when Mildred was acting matron, CCS No. 2 admitted almost 41,000 sick and wounded soldiers, of whom approximately 1,200 died, and its medical staff performed almost 7,500 operations.[13]

On March 21, 1918, German troops launched a major spring offensive, pushing back the Allies and wreaking havoc on the medical system. CCS No. 2, due to "heavy shelling in this area," closed temporarily on March 18,[14] sending its nursing staff to St. Omer for safety. They returned on March 29, only to be evacuated again on only half an hour's notice on April 14. Mildred's letters remain remarkably upbeat during this period, despite the dangers. The CCS re-opened 25 kilometres west, at Esquelbecq, and began receiving patients on April 26.

Mildred and Laura remained with CCS No. 2 until August 22, 1918,[15] when Mildred voluntarily resigned her matronship. During that month, the Canadians had acted as shock troops in the Battle of Amiens farther south, pushing the Germans back. This victory heralded the beginning of the end of the war.[16] Matron-in-Chief Macdonald allowed the two friends to choose their next posting, and they decided on the peace of the much smaller Canadian Forestry Corps Hospital in the Jura district of France, near the Swiss mountains, well away from the battlefields. Six weeks later, transferred to the newly established Forestry Corps hospital at Facture, near Bordeaux,[17] they were plunged into the epidemic of influenza that eventually killed more people than had been killed during the war. The war ended on November 11, 1918, but Laura and Mildred's nursing work continued into 1919. After the dangers and stresses of 1917 and 1918, it is a relief to know that they spent a delightful leave on the Riviera in January 1919, albeit plagued by yet another officious British administrator.

Laura and Mildred sailed for Canada and home on May 7, 1919, after almost four years with the CAMC.

> No. 2 Canadian Casualty
> Clearing Station
> [Remy Siding]
> July 27th, 1917

My dear Cairine,

I wonder if you are all down at St. Andrews. How I would love to walk in upon you! But just now I am leading rather a different life than the lovely peaceful kind you have....

Of course it is almost useless to write letters for there is very little we can say – though I could *tell* you a great deal.[18]

Lollie & I came up here nearly two weeks ago. We had a day in London, which was welcome as there were a lot of small things we wanted to see to, a last final shampoo, etc. Then at Boulogne we were lucky enough to have an extra day. We paid [a visit to] the much talked of (in Montreal) McGill Unit.[19] They have a very nice place there, though I am very pleased I am not with them.

We like it very much here. The work is hard but one has the satisfaction of feeling we are doing something. We have a very shifting population, as we don't keep the patients for more than 24 hours, except for exceptional cases.

One realizes the horrors of war more than ever in this place. We can only hope that it will soon be over.

This camp is so nice – it is very well laid out & splendidly run. The grounds are very attractive, as we have a Sergeant who is a landscape gardener,

& the place is certainly a credit to him. We have heaps of sweet peas, nasturtiums, morning glories [&] violas, & all so well laid out.

Our quarters are very comfortable. We have the same kind of canvas huts as we had in the East. Of course it is so much more civilized here than in Salonika – not to speak of Lemnos – that one hasn't the same feeling at all about "active service."

At present Lollie & I are on night duty, a necessary evil, though I don't really mind it here except for the lack of sleep. Three hours in the day is my maximum, & that soon makes one feel rather tired & "nervy." However we only have it for four weeks. Most nights I am so busy that I don't have time to feel sleepy.[20]

I am on the Officer's ward & don't mind it. As a matter of fact, most people rather want to avoid it, but here [the Officers] are easily satisfied. It is all by way of comparison, & it seems very comfortable here to them. It really is a very nice hut, with canvas on the walls & polished linoleum on [the] floor.

The mosquitoes are very large & hungry here – people get fearful bites.

We are both flourishing & know the life will be a healthy one as we are out in the open air so much.

I feel this is a very stupid letter, but it is hard being tied down. It gives one a feeling of having nothing to say.

...

> With love to you all. Affect. Yours.
> Mildred H. Forbes.

> No. 2 CCS
> August 29th, 1917

My dear Cairine,

Today we were discussing Xmas, which though far off still, we have got to think of ... as it takes a long time to get parcels ... up to us.

Miss Graham, who is in charge of this C.C.S,[21] is leaving shortly, & alas I have got to take her place – though I shall never be able to fill it. The thought of it does not please me particularly. Still, Miss Macdonald has been at me for some position, so this is the easiest way out of it.

Well, this is rather far off my subject. What I started to say was Miss Graham said last year the Canadian Red Cross played them false, & had it not been for individual boxes, the patients & Men of the Unit would have come off very badly. It does seem to me a shame that the C.S.Ss should not get lots, for here we are getting the Men straight from the trenches, & it does seem to me that here of all places they should spend as happy a Xmas as possible. It occurred to me that perhaps the Rockland Red Cross might be inclined to send us either some stockings (Xmas) or anything of that type for Xmas. Of course I know you have your own Rockland Men to look after, but I thought ... the ladies might be interested in working for some special object as well, for sometimes people prefer to do that rather than hand their stuff into the general stock to be sent off anywhere. However don't feel *obliged* to take this up, for you probably have more than you can do there.

Lollie is going to write her Mother, who is a keen worker in the I.O.D.E., & get her circle to send us stuff as well for Xmas, for we probably will have about 400 people to see to at Xmas – that includes our own Canadian personnel of the Unit.

It is so cold & bleak & rainy at present that everyone feels blue. The weather is hard on the men. They come in soaked through & through, & they are so caked with mud that they are about unrecognizable.

I am off night duty, & am on the officers' ward at present. In a few days' time I come off to go on with Miss Graham to get on to the ropes of running the place. Under ordinary circumstances there are nine sisters here, but this summer for obvious reasons we are thirty-two.[22]

I wonder if you are all at St. Andrews. It seems so far away & sounds so peaceful & safe. I often wonder if Lollie & I will get home intact. It is a pretty hot spot at times – though I have never told my family so – but I so often worry in case any thing should happen to Lollie, for her Mother's sake chiefly.[23] Luckily her Mother is not worrying, for she has no idea where we are. Well we all have to take our chance, & when one sees the splendid Men thrown away, one feels why should we value our lives? I have a young officer here, only 24, who is an organist who has just had his right arm amputated. I shall never forget his utter misery when he was told. One sees so many tragedies all the time that one feels positively sick.

Well, my letter is not very cheerful – please excuse the scrawl.

Much love to you all.
Mildred H Forbes

No. 2 CCS
October 11th, 1917

My dear Cairine,

It seems a long time since I have seen your familiar writing, but I expect you have been having a busy time settling your family for the Autumn after St. Andrews.

How I would like to drop in to see you all at Rockland. I expect you are beginning to get colder weather now, & Norman's river will soon be freezing.[24]

Talk about cold! It feels like a sharp November day, & you know living in tents & canvas huts with huge cracks in them is chilly work. Still we *can* get warm – which is more than the poor Men in the line can do. Their sufferings are awful. We have had such wet weather the last week or so ... that they are never dry. The thought of the winter is appalling.

Bob Moyse[25] was here yesterday – his regiment are somewhere in the vicinity. He evidently is a friend of one of the sisters here, & he came to tea. The minute I saw him & heard his name of course I recognized him....

We have been *very* busy, but all the news is so very encouraging, everyone is feeling very pleased.

The Men are simply wonderful. The people at home have *no idea* what the soldiers are going through for them. I feel it would not do for me to go home before the war is over, for after what I have seen here, I feel that I would make many enemies by my remarks to the stay-at-homes. However if conscription ever gets going properly, these people will see some of it, though the conscripts will find they have a lot to live down when they meet the Men who have been in it for three years.

Well, I am beginning to rant so must stop – but really the sights here are enough to break one's heart.

With Much love to you all.

Affect. Yours.
Mildred H. Forbes

No. 2 CCS
November 20th, 1917

My dear Cairine,

Four very well filled stockings have arrived already, and I am simply delighted to hear the others are on their way. I am afraid it has given you and the Rockland Red Cross people a great deal of trouble. I cannot thank you enough for these things, & I know they will be very much appreciated.

It is so hard to plan for Xmas, for so many of the sisters who are now here will probably not be with us later, & they cannot take the same interest.

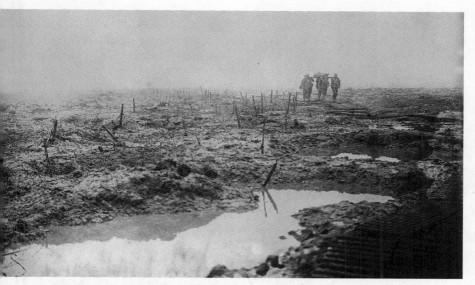

Canadian stretcher bearers bringing wounded through mud, Battle of Passchendaele, November 1917. *Canada, Dept. of National Defence/Library and Archives Canada PA-002367*

One of the girls, a Miss Boultbee[26] from B.C. who is quite a friend of ours & particularly nice, gave me £5 to use – some money which had been sent to her. So we are expending that on decorations. We sent in a large order to Dennison's the paper people, so I feel the huts will look well anyway.

We have our chickens for the patients & Men's dinner – we are fattening them up. We are now puzzling our brains as to what we shall get for the Men of the Unit. Last year the Officers & Sisters gave them a portable billiard table which pleased them very much.

One has to think so far ahead that it is somewhat hard to plan.

We continue to be quite busy, & we are now undergoing some rather trying changes – a new O.C. & several other officers. In bygone days, they had some very good people in this Unit, & it is hard to see the place going downhill.

We enjoyed having the Canadians up here so much, & certainly they did some splendid work. We have every reason to be proud of our Men, for certainly they do things that the others find impossible.[27]

Our Mess was always crowded at tea time. I met Major O'Connor[28] of Ottawa – he was in a couple of times with General C.[29] We have such long conversations about Ottawa.

Teddie Savage[30] I saw several times. He looks very well & is really a striking looking figure.

I also saw Wilfred Bovey & Ned Fetherstonhaugh.[31] The latter looks very thin & worn. Prince Arthur of C[onnaught][32] also came & had tea with us.

It was really nice seeing a few Canadians, but now we are desolate again.

Am hoping to have a visit from the Matron in Chief shortly. I will be so glad to see her as I have so many points to go over with her.

...

It is remarkably mild here at present. I only hope it lasts.

We had our third case of diptheria develop among the Sisters. We cannot trace the cause at all. It is a great worry.

...

Rockland seems so frightfully far away. We talk of the days when the war is over & we can all get home, but it all seems so hopeless.

There are so many really badly off & losing all they possess that I feel ashamed complaining.

My notepaper is rather pathetic – some provided by the Red X for the patients.

With love to you all & best wishes for Christmas & the New Year.

> Affect. yours
> Mildred H. Forbes

No. 2 CCS
January 3rd, 1918

My dear Cairine,

The six cases reached us on New Year's Day & if you could only have seen the delight of the men who received the stockings, you would have felt more than repaid for all the trouble you have taken.

At first we were heart-broken that none of our cases from Canada arrived in time for Xmas, but really now I have decided that it was a good thing they were late, for we were able to give pleasure to so many more men.

About a week before Xmas we abandoned all hope of seeing your boxes & Mrs. Holland's eight, so we sisters set to work & made 300 stockings out of mosquito netting. We visited Colonel Blaylock at B. & grabbed everything we could to fill the stockings.[33] Some of the girls had had money sent them, so we purchased a lot of odds & ends. We then split up the stockings you had sent by mail & used some things that Mary Thompson's circle had sent.

In the end the stockings were well filled & certainly they delighted the men.

You see in a C.C.S. we don't keep our patients long. Those that can travel only stay in about 12 [to] 24 hours, so that by the time New Year's came, we had an entirely different lot of men who had not had a bit of Xmas. Really I have never seen children more delighted than these men were with their stockings. When I went into the tent, the men were lying very dejectedly in the darkness. When the stockings appeared, they bucked right up and their pleasure was a sight to behold. I really had so much pleasure in seeing these poor souls so happy.

I will write a more formal note for the Red Cross Society, and I hope they will realize how much their contributions were appreciated. My stocking was splendid – thanks so much for the smokes.

The Men had a splendid Xmas dinner – very good chickens, plum pudding, mince tarts, tomato soup, etc., etc.

One old Scotchman who is being kept as a duty patient said "never in his life had he spent such a happy Xmas" & he added "the worst of it is I cannot tell you how much I enjoyed it" & he promptly burst into tears!

The Men have such a hard life here & do without so much that the simplest thing pleases them. Poor souls they are just about being frozen now. It is bitterly cold.

All we sisters are hobbling about with chilblains. Everyone is borrowing larger boots. It is a terrible business.

I hope that you all had a Happy Xmas. I am sure the children must have enjoyed themselves.

With much love to you all & many thanks for all your work in connection with the stockings.

> Affect. Yours.
> Mildred.

> No. 2 CCS
> February 12th, 1918

My dear Cairine,

I was more than delighted to get your letter.... It was such a treat hearing all the news of your doings ... and the rest of your family. It really was quite like a tonic to me, for we get so fed up with this abnormal life we are leading.

As a matter of fact, both Lollie & I are happier here than we could be anywhere else in the Service, for this C.C.S. is such a nice one – and certainly we are lucky in the girls who are up here with us.

Hope Wurtele's sister Rhoda is here.[34] She is a particularly nice girl....

It has been such a mild winter that we are very lucky, for the misery everyone endures when it is cold is beyond everything.

The men of the Unit have been very busy getting up a concert party. It promises to be a great success. We have been having a great time getting up their Pierrot suits. They asked us to make them! Poor Lollie has been shouldering all the responsibility, as you know how much I sew! Last night they had their first dress rehearsal, which Lollie & I attended. It really is going to be a wonderfully good show.

I wonder if you ever see that illustrated paper "Canada." They had a few pictures of a C.C.S. in France in December & January. If you get a chance have a look at them ... they are pictures we had taken last summer, & which we are unable to send through the mail.

A week ago I had a great shock in hearing of Kenneth's sudden death.[35] Of course you know the worry he has been from time to time. Apparently he was acting rather badly for the past year, & the family could do nothing for him. It is pathetic what drink will do. He was taken suddenly ill & died at the Montreal General Hospital.

He had a wretched life, and yet there seemed so little one could do.

I felt very badly ... though it was hardly a personal loss, as I had seen so little of Kenneth. Yet when one feels it is one's own flesh & blood, & then when one sees splendid men dying over here for us all, it seems such a disgrace to think of an able bodied man dying at home from drink. It certainly is a terrible curse.

Well – it is no good harrowing you too much!

With much love to you all. Affect. yrs.
   Mildred.

[P.S.] ...

At 9:30 a.m. on 14 April, CCS No. 2 abruptly closed down operations at Remy Siding due to heavy shelling and was ordered to Esquelbecq, about 15 miles from Dunkirk. The nurses were sent to British CCS No. 13 at Arnèke, rejoining their own CCS in Esquelbecq on 18 April and billetted in the village. CCS No. 2 began admitting patients on the 26th. Formerly in huts, the CCS was now in tents.[36]

No. 2 CCS
[Esquelbecq]
April 25th, 1918

My dear Cairine,

The lovely box of chocolates arrived today. Thanks so much for them. They were very welcome, & are so nice & fresh.

I received a letter from you a few days ago, but we have been rather on the move & have mislaid it. The Arabs are not in it with us these days.

We are in such a pretty part of the country just now, really nicer than our other situation, but this does not feel like home! Everything was so well planned & comfortable before.

I am glad to say we are living in billets rather than tents & are really most comfortable. Lollie & I have a very nice room – our own camp beds, wash stand made out of Red Cross boxes, but have a handsome mantle piece, [&] a cupboard & a wardrobe with long pier glass!! Such style I have not lived in for a long time.

You would be amused if you could have seen us last week when we were temporarily attached to a British C.C.S. They were very kind to us. Thirteen of us landed in & they put us in a large hut which had previously been used by wounded refugees. They left some of their livestock, which rather took to us![37] Otherwise we were quite happy.... It was the simple life. We amused ourselves by sleeping, eating, and going for walks. Reading was almost out of the question as someone was always talking somewhere near! I was glad when the order came to rejoin our Unit.

The season seems so well advanced it is hard to realize it is only April. I expect things are beginning to come on with you.

Excuse this scrawl. I am writing in bed, as it is 10:30 p.m. & I retire early.

Much love to you all
    Affect Yours. Mildred

No. 2 CCS
June 25th, 1918

My dear Cairine,

The parcel containing cigarettes and the stockings arrived safely three days ago. Very many thanks for the smokes. They are most acceptable. Of course the stockings are a perfect delight to me, for it is practically impossible to get tan stockings in England, & as we always wear them, one's feet get to be a worry. Last Xmas Muriel sent me some Holeproof lisle stockings – but for them I would have nothing to wear. Last time I saw Miss Macdonald I suggested that she would have to make a change & allow us to wear black footwear, for though I dislike black with blue cotton dresses, it gets to be a fearful problem how we are to get tan boots.

A friend of Edith Wilson's is with this Unit – a Miss Domville.[38] I wonder what she is like to meet socially, for she seems an odd character to me.

We are not very busy now, & at present I am suffering from stiffness from taking vigorous exercise. Ring tennis is a great amusement for all ranks. We use a rubber ring made of tubing. It is the same game as they play on shipboard. I would far rather have the real tennis, but at present that seems impossible.

We had to send Rhoda Wurtele down to the Base sick last week. She had an attack of Trench Fever, & as it takes some time to get fit again, we had to send her off. She will likely get to England & have some sick leave.

I was sorry to see her go, for she is a particularly nice girl, far superior to her sister – *Lady* Tupper's friend![39]

This is a very pretty part of the country. Of course all under cultivation. It seems queer to see hay being cut in June. The fields are a sight just now.

Last Saturday Lollie & I went to D[unkirk][40] partly on pleasure & business. I was really in search of a laundry for the sisters' clothes. From time to time we have to change, owing to the *war*,[41] & now we are not near many towns large enough to possess a steam laundry.

The country folk about here do not go in much for good washing, & we wear so many starched things – collars, cuffs, veils, etc. – that I find a large laundry more satisfactory. We managed to get what we wanted at a sea side place. We went to the shore but there was a strong wind blowing & the sand sifting about everywhere.

Last week I had quite a week of trips as I took Miss Wurtele to St. O[mer],[42] her first stopping place on her journey. The Medical Officer, rather a decent sort, came down in the ambulance too, so after we had left the patient, we proceeded to have a very nice lunch.

The strawberries were lovely that day.

It is now nearly a year since Lollie & I came to this Unit, & I am sure any day we will have to leave. I will be sorry to leave this place though glad to give up my Matronship, even if it does mean forfeiting my pay. I certainly have not earned my £30 a month. Still in comparison with others in the Army, I suppose I have done as much as many others who are getting twice that amount.

I wonder if this will find you at St. Andrews....

Well I feel I have ambled on at great length – without much news.
With Much love to you all & hoping you are all well.

> Affect. yours.
> Mildred

No. 2 CCS
July 24th, 1918

My dear Cairine,

The box of chocolates arrived in splendid condition & we are enjoying
them so much. Very many thanks. I assure you they are a very great treat.
I also received a letter from you written the week before you left for St.
Andrews.

I expect you are all enjoying that place now. It is wonderful to think of
you all being able to motor without having to worry about the lack of petrol.

I don't really see why you should feel ashamed about getting a new car.
By doing so you are keeping business going. Also you are doing your part
in your own line. I assure you I think the people slaving at home doing Red
Cross work are certainly doing their share.

... Personally I feel I have been lucky in getting over here, though one gets
very fed up at times.

I am afraid many of us are going to be changed so much that ordinary
existence is going to be very trying. We have seen such tremendous things
going on that trifles at home are going to seem very petty.

Wasn't it *awful* about those fourteen girls on the Hospital ship? I knew
most of them & it haunts me at night. The Canadian girls have been paying
the price lately.[43]

We had a most successful visit from Miss Macdonald (the Matron in
Chief) & her Canadian Representative in France. They came one afternoon
& spent the night. All went very well. I always enjoy seeing Miss Macdonald,
though I felt rather worried as this was their first visit to our new camp.
However they approved very much of everything.

Holland & I are to leave as soon as the new Matron comes to take my
place. We are going down to the Canadian Forestry Hospital in the south.
It is in the Jura district. I was asked where we wanted to go, & I thought it
would be nice to have a distinct change. After a year at a C.C.S. something
fairly peaceful appeals to me, though it might be tiresome after a while.

...

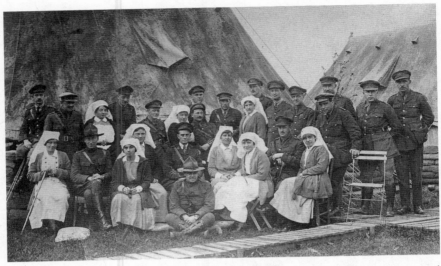

Staff, Casualty Clearing Station No. 2. Laura stands to centre right, her body turned towards Mildred, who sits just left of Laura. *From the personal photo album of Nursing Sister Clare Gass*

I had a nice letter from Anna[44] the other day. She seems to be settled in Sunningdale, [England]. She gave us both an invitation to go & stay with her. How I wish we could! One longs for a comfortable civilized life. However I have no leave due me so I cannot get away.

I do hope this odd assortment of notepaper won't disturb you, & that you won't open this in front of some of your stylish friends. I happen to be out of notepaper, so have to use "scraps."

Much love to you all.

Affect. yours.
Mildred

No. 2 CCS
August 21st, 1918

My dear Cairine,

...

This is my last day at No. 2 C.C.S. & I feel very sorry to leave the place. Miss Squire[45] is taking my job over. She is a very nice girl, & just the one for the position.

We leave by ambulance for B[oulogne] tomorrow morning & then go on the next day to Paris en route to the Jura. It will be a long tiresome trip. I only wish that we might stay off in Paris for a few days, but am afraid that as we are not due leave ... we will have to go right through.

Everyone says that it is lovely down in the Jura. It ought to be lovely country as it is so near Switzerland.

Will write soon again but today have only time for a short note. With much love to you all.

Affect. yours
Mildred

Canadian Forestry Corps
Hospital
Jura Mountains
October 4th, 1918

My dear Cairine,

I seem to have received so many things from you lately, all of which were very welcome.

First came a letter from St Andrews, date unknown, as I am writing this on duty. It was the day you had entertained my illustrious relatives the Galts.

Then came a box of cigarettes, most acceptable, & the tan stockings – of course all the greatest treat. Very many thanks for them. It is simply impossible to get even half decent tan stockings in England, so I now feel very set up.

A lovely box of chocolates arrived about two days ago from you. We are enjoying them so much & eat them very carefully & slowly – thanks so much for them.

Well – isn't the war news splendid?[46] I hate to be here in this "safety first" spot when everyone is so busy nearer the front. Here we only have sick & accidents from the Forestry Corps, & while I realize the Men are doing most important work for the Army, still one does feel side tracked. We are fairly busy, as many of the Men have pneumonia & such troubles, but it is a very inconvenient Hospital, so that when one goes to do the slightest thing, there is a huge commotion. It all seems so futile after a busy place.

We have done quite a little sight-seeing during our free time. Lollie & I went up to Besançon last Sunday afternoon by train & spent Monday there. It is a very interesting town, & I was only sorry that we could not have remained longer, for besides the interest of the place, the hotel was really quite comfortable. I was anxious to stay on, but of course had to come back.

By the way, my movements are very uncertain so will you address letters still to 133 Oxford St. as they will always forward them on.

It is getting quite cold here, but the country is looking lovely. This is a hurried scrawl on awful paper, but I wanted to send a line off to tell you how much I appreciated your kindness.

I hope you & the family & Norman are all flourishing. Give them all my love & keep a share for yourself.

> Affect. Yours.
> Mildred.

Did I tell you we had dined at Lady Wurtele-MacDougall's.[47] She is much the same – she has a dear little boy, very spoilt, but nice in spite of it. I am sorry for hubby!

> Canadian Forestry Hospital
> 12th District
> October 31st, 1918

My dear Cairine,

I was delighted to receive your letter of September 29th a few days ago. Your hands must be more than full I should think, and now that you are expecting a small Angus,[48] I do hope you will try & take life fairly easy.

Thank goodness for a few weeks in December. You will be *forced* to stay in bed so that you may have a little rest, for I am sure you need it. By the time I get home, your family will be grown up.... I hope that the newest one may be not too old before I meet him!

I am sure you will be glad in many respects to be in Ottawa this winter.[49] It will relieve you a great deal to have the children at school. It seems hard to realize they have got to that stage.

The Rockland people will miss you terribly.... But I am awfully glad for your sake you will have a change.

Of course just what was Mackenzie[50] ... talking about regarding my desirable position in the C.A.M.C.? He must be crazy.

I was Matron while at the C.C.S., & I confess No. 2 was the best C.C.S. in the C.A.M.C. & it had a good reputation. But when my time was up there, I relinquished my Matronship voluntarily, as I was tired of that type of work.

The Forestry Hospital in the Jura was a small affair, & I went down as an ordinary Nursing Sister. After being there six weeks, orders came for Lollie & myself & one other to go to the 12th District Canadian Forestry Camp near Bordeaux[51] to start a Hospital there, & here we are. I am nominally in charge, but it is no very magnificent job, though we quite like the place. Unfortunately we landed here in the midst of a fearful epidemic of influenza, & we have been rushed ever since.[52]

I wired immediately for a fourth Sister, & we have been worked fearfully hard. The cases have been terrible & the deaths appalling. Our Senior Medical Officer has been taken to Bordeaux to the American Hospital with the flu, & we cannot but wonder if we are going to be able to escape ourselves. The last few days the cases have been somewhat less severe, so we are hoping that perhaps the epidemic may be on the wane.

We have really had little chance of seeing the country. I motored up to Bordeaux one day on a shopping expedition to procure necessaries for our Mess. It struck me as being a lovely place, & I hope to go back when I have more leisure.

There is a very attractive seaside place called Arcachon about 15 miles from here. I went down yesterday with the laundry. Apparently quite a lot of French people go there in the winter. It seemed odd to see children playing in the sand & wading in October.

If this epidemic ever ends, we ought to quite enjoy the country, though it seems very flat in this immediate vicinity & ugly after the Jura Mountains.

We have rooms in a French house. It is a funny little bungalow shaped place, built by peasants. It was a pity that they took these quarters for us instead of building us a hut in the Hospital grounds.

The Major who made these arrangements before we came is a nice, kind old woman, who hasn't much business head. He had agreed with the Frenchwoman that she would cook for us, but she had absolutely no idea of cooking & was filthy dirty. We stood her for a week, then I went & said we had to have an Army cook. We have one now installed so we are getting some food.

We just have two bedrooms & a livingroom where we have our meals, & a kitchen. It is small, but we are not off much except in the evenings & then we are glad to go to bed fairly early.

The days are nice & warm. The sun is positively hot. The nights are terribly cold, however, & one needs loads of blankets. The Jaegar blankets I got from you have been such a comfort. I could not have existed without them.

You will be tired of reading this scrawl – so I must stop.

With love to you all.
    Affect. yours.
      Mildred

Canadian Forestry Hospital,
12th District
January 25th, 1919[53]

My dear Cairine,

    Upon my return from leave I found your letter awaiting me. I was delighted to hear of the arrival of Miss ? Wilson,[54] & that all was well over for Xmas. You are certainly the right person to have babies, for they are always so good & well behaved! When I think of the fuss & ceremony over young Mildred Hope![55]

...

    How glad I was to hear that you were in Ottawa this winter. It will be such a nice change after Rockland, & I am sure you will be thankful on the children's account.

    We enjoyed our leave on the Riviera so much. Of course the warm sunny days & brightness appealed to us so much after mud & living more & less uncomfortably for over three years.

    One of the chief joys of leave to me is the baths! One gets so tired of bathing in a quart of water.

    We broke our journey very well coming home, taking a little extra time, as we have good natured people at this end. At the best of times it is an awkward journey from Bordeaux.... We spent one night at Marseilles & left there at midday for Avignon, where we had from 3 p.m. till 9 a.m. the following day. It is such a lovely old place. I only wished we could have remained there longer. We went further homeward & then spent the next night at Carcassone. I wonder if you ever have seen that quaint old walled city, marred only by its filth & smells! I noticed some Hun officers imprisoned in the Chateau & was delighted to realize how uncomfortable they must be there. It is a good place for them.

    I had previously wired our O.C. that we would be arriving in ... Bordeaux by the evening train, & ... a car came up to meet us. Our little house looked quite cozy & homelike when we got back. I must say I was not looking forward particularly to returning here after our leave; however, it is a nice rest!! There is very little work at present, as the influenza seems to be quiet once more. The Forestry people are more or less marking time till they can return to Canada.

I don't believe I have told you about the wonderful house we were staying in during our leave at ... Roquebrune. A Mrs. Angus, an Australian, rented the house as a sort of club for overseas Sisters. It is a beautiful house owned by a very rich Irish man who made his money in cement. The house itself is quite noted, & it certainly seemed like a palace to us with its huge marble halls & beautiful furniture. Can you imagine sleeping in an inlaid bed after using a camp bed for ages? The gardens were lovely, though the lawns which *were* renowned were all cabbages owing to the war. Still, the roses & orange & lemon trees were there – one garden went right down to the beach. It certainly was a gorgeous spot, only marred by silly rules & regulations made & enforced by a prim Matron who glared at us severely! However in *spite* of her we enjoyed ourselves, though I must say it is a rest returning to duty where we do what we want!!!

...

Much love to you all. Mildred.

Conclusion and Epilogue

Canadian First World War military nurses are deemed to have "more symbolic than historical value,"[1] but remembering them as "ministering angels"[2] and "bluebirds" erases the nurses' "actual [wartime] work."[3] Such sanctified images also erase the women themselves: their personalities, their attitudes, and their complexities. The letters of Laura Holland and Mildred Forbes help reclaim military nurses' lives, work, and methods of coping with war. Their words vividly depict four years dedicated to nursing ill and wounded soldiers, sometimes under trying conditions. They also reveal modern, determined women who enjoyed cocktails, adventure, laughter, and music and who were unafraid to speak out on behalf of themselves and their patients. Certainly the two were privileged, both socially and professionally, in part because of Mildred's close relationship with Matron-in-Chief Macdonald. But like their fellow nurses, they would have laughed at the thought of themselves as "angels."

Such images, too, suppress the "radical implications" of women's work[4] by "focusing on the needs of the nation, particularly its soldiers."[5] Envisioning nurses as "ministering angels" stifles their sexuality and their risky proximity to the male body.[6] As well, during the war, much public discourse translated dead and wounded soldiers into Christ-like, self-sacrificial heroes, thus glorifying or hiding their "bloody bod[ies]" to create meaningful deaths.[7] Laura's and Mildred's letters, written to trusted female correspondents, expose both pitiful male bodies and the neglect of men; such witnessing could be far more dangerous to the war effort than sexuality.

On Lemnos, Laura and Mildred linked the dead, ill, and dying soldiers to the British administration's incompetence. For Laura, the term "sacrifice" became the equivalent of "slaughter": men were sacrificed not for a cause, but because of the "ignorance, & in-capability of many" of the administrative "heads."[8] Forbes, too, revealed the inhumanity of war, telling of a soldier who, "when his comrade was dying beside him ... was not *allowed* to give him a drink of water – for it has to be kept for the well people who will live. Doesn't it seem awful?"[9] Mildred depicts the military as indifferent and neglectful, responsible for the "awful ... conditions" of the trenches and the subsequent illnesses of the soldiers she tends.[10] Instead of wounded heroes injured in battle, these patients are reduced to "wrecks" and "pathetic sights," victims of their own commanders and administrators.[11] The nurses reveal men dying of illness and in want, in an ironic reversal of the "supreme sacrifice" of popular discourse.

Sharing these stories with Mrs. Holland and Cairine Wilson was a means of trying to help the patients. Because of the shortages, the nurses were unable to supply even the bare necessities for their patients, and this problem reflected on their professional reputations. "The Canadian Hospitals in France seem to have made a wonderful name for themselves ... from the patients['] point of [view]," Holland wrote to her mother, "but ... we are not making any such impression here."[12] The work of the women at home became of national importance; by sending supplies, those at home would contribute to Canada's reputation abroad. The military and public discourses of the time privileged battle wounds over illness. Because many of their patients were ill with dysentery and other enteric diseases, Laura and Mildred persuasively emphasized the soldiers' trench and battle experiences, creating causal connections between trench conditions, illness, and neglect. For instance, Holland described one soldier who "had been @ the Peninsula for five months, & for the past three had *never* been out of the trenches once, but had been on duty 2 hrs. & off 2 hrs. night & day for all that time – then he comes here with pleurisy, & we can give him *so little*. Do you wonder we feel there is mis-management somewhere[?]"[13] Such stories had influence, as the constant boxes of supplies from home testified.

But this exposure of soldiers' bodies made ill due to incompetence was contested ground for the nurses. Paradoxically, their gender both protected them and exposed them to critique. Nurses, as women, were supposed to be protected and safe from harm. The deaths of a nurse and the matron of CSH No. 3 from dysentery, combined with details of the water shortage, food shortages, and harsh conditions that the nurses worked under on Lemnos, caused an uproar that the deaths of men from the same illness did not. An official inspection of the hospitals was held, better food was provided, and conditions did improve; the nurses' complaints and letters home, some to influential families, had worked.[14] Yet the nurses were accused of leaking information, characterized as gossips, and threatened with severe censorship, which was seen as affecting only the "*Canadian* letters."[15] Censorship was a constant theme in Laura's letters. It threatened her close relationship with her mother, and it also jeopardized her patients, because her mother's home group had become an essential source of patient supplies. Laura mostly honoured the prohibition on military information, but she saw little sense in eliminating descriptions of hospital life and her own living conditions. Other nurses may have seen "silence" and "a willingness to die for the Empire" as ways to become "good soldiers."[16] Laura pragmatically skewered such tenets, seeing no need to "die for the Empire" (or suffer for it) because of others' shoddy administrative work. Continuing to write also meant rejecting characterizations of female nurses as silent and submissive. Laura did not appropriate or adhere to a masculine "soldier's code"; instead, she created her own notions of a nurse's duty and responsibility. To remain silent was to neglect patients; to speak was to care for patients and to protect the nurses' own health.

In a different context, self-sacrifice did become acceptable. When Mildred was acting matron of CCS No. 2 in France, with Laura a nursing sister, death from shelling and air raids was a constant threat.[17] Mildred made nurses and soldiers, women and men, equal, commenting that "we all have to take our chance, & when one sees the splendid Men thrown away, one feels why should we value our lives"?[18] To her, women should not be privileged or protected. She continued by describing "a young officer here ... who is an organist who has just had his right arm amputated. I shall never forget his utter misery when he was told."[19] From her position of power, untroubled by censorship regulations, Mildred related a story she would have been forbidden to tell on Lemnos – and she told it in terms of "misery" instead of the expected terms of stoicism. Her patient was not a hero with glorious wounds, but a young man who had lost his profession and his calling because of war. Mildred saw beyond death and its supposed glory: the men "thrown away" were not just the dead, but those who must live on, mutilated or disabled. Tellingly, Mildred was quite willing to give up her own life, but "I so often worry in case anything should happen to [Laura]."[20]

Laura, too, demonstrated her growing realization of the gendered value of her training and work. She commented, for instance, that "you only had to see a hospital run entirely by men to realize how much better things went where there are women."[21] Later, she repeatedly reinforced the distinction between genders: "If the War has taught me one thing it is that certain work can only be properly done by women, & other work by men. Of course the difficult point to decide, & over which the both sexes would have many arguments, is just which part *is* a woman's work, & which part a man's."[22] She rejected the concept that the nurses, rather than the orderlies, should perform routine cleaning tasks, [23] instead considering the nurses better qualified than either male officers or orderlies to design the organization and set up of hospital wards in new postings.[24] Laura's perspective demonstrates that military nurses, aware of their value to the military, could and did rebel against male authority.

In their years of friendship and war work, Laura and Mildred had only one documented disagreement: Laura bought eggs for her patients on Lemnos out of her own salary, and Mildred declared that she didn't "approve."[25] Mildred was speaking from the perspective of an administrator who felt that better organization should obtain eggs for all of the men, not just some of them; Laura was acting from the perspective of a nurse who wanted to change the monotonous, scant diet her men were being fed. Throughout the war years, Mildred appeared to be the professional leader, but Laura's actions in this case showed her independence and her willingness to act on her own beliefs. The friendship, from their letters, flowed smoothly for the rest of the war. Laura did feel that it was endangered when Matron-in-Chief Macdonald recommended her for the Royal Red Cross for her work in the Mediterranean, but withheld Mildred's till a later date. Mildred, as the more experienced nurse, could have felt threatened by her friend's award; instead, she insisted on sending a telegram to Laura's family, "shower[ed] [her] with attentions," and suppressed any personal disappointment she might have felt.[26] Laura declared that she would "never quite forgive" Miss Macdonald for separating the pair so that Mildred could not share the experience of the Investiture.[27] Clearly, Laura felt what she did not say: that Miss Macdonald had deliberately created a situation that could have damaged the friendship, an unforgivable sin.

Laura and Mildred's friendship became much more than the "common interests and tastes" that usually "link" friends.[28] They had survived the tensions of Lemnos and the chaos of the CCS, cared for one another through debilitating illnesses, thoroughly enjoyed exploring their exotic locations, and overcome professional tensions; they had lived in overcrowded tents, huts, and rooms for four years, yet had created homes for and with one another, never seeming to tire of one another's company. And they had worked together, sometimes as equals, at other times with Laura subordinate to her friend's authority. Part of their loyalty to one another was also their loyalty to the demands of nursing during wartime: if Mildred was in charge of the work and the morale of CCS No. 2, Laura actively and wholeheartedly shared in creating the "best CCS in the C.A.M.C,"[29] their common goal being to make whole the wounded and ill soldiers who filled the beds. Both learned from the communal tensions on Lemnos and at Salonika; when they reached the CCS in France, they expanded the tiny, safe "home" they had created to the nurses and male medical staff they were responsible for, creating community and comradeship in the midst of war.

EPILOGUE

Laura Holland and Mildred Forbes's remarkable friendship endured beyond the war. Discharged in May 1919, they left nursing to study social welfare at Boston's Simmons College, graduating in 1920.[30] Both accepted positions at Montreal General Hospital, with Mildred in charge of the new Social Service Department of Public Health,[31] and Laura a social service worker.[32] Unfortunately, the illnesses that Mildred had suffered during the war "left their marks upon [her] constitution."[33] Hospitalized in December 1920, Mildred Forbes, RRC, Médaille des epidémies en argent, mentioned in despatches, died on January 13, 1921,[34] a late war casualty.

Laura Holland, bereft of her friend, left Montreal for Toronto in 1921, accepting the position of Director of Nursing and Emergency Department of

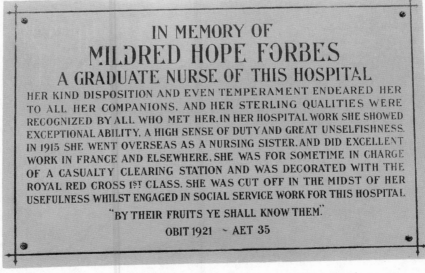

IN MEMORY OF
MILDRED HOPE FORBES
A GRADUATE NURSE OF THIS HOSPITAL

HER KIND DISPOSITION AND EVEN TEMPERAMENT ENDEARED HER TO ALL HER COMPANIONS, AND HER STERLING QUALITIES WERE RECOGNIZED BY ALL WHO MET HER. IN HER HOSPITAL WORK SHE SHOWED EXCEPTIONAL ABILITY, A HIGH SENSE OF DUTY AND GREAT UNSELFISHNESS. IN 1915 SHE WENT OVERSEAS AS A NURSING SISTER. AND DID EXCELLENT WORK IN FRANCE AND ELSEWHERE, SHE WAS FOR SOMETIME IN CHARGE OF A CASUALTY CLEARING STATION AND WAS DECORATED WITH THE ROYAL RED CROSS 1ST CLASS. SHE WAS CUT OFF IN THE MIDST OF HER USEFULNESS WHILST ENGAGED IN SOCIAL SERVICE WORK FOR THIS HOSPITAL

"BY THEIR FRUITS YE SHALL KNOW THEM."

OBIT 1921 ~ AET 35

Plaque in memory of Mildred Forbes, Montreal General Hospital. *Alumnae Association of the Montreal General Hospital School of Nursing* the Ontario Division of the Red Cross Society, [35] and appointed Superintendent of the Ontario Division of the Red Cross in 1922.[36] During this time, she organized the first Red Cross outpost hospitals in Wilberforce, Haileybury, and Englehart,[37] small hospitals staffed by one or two nurses that "supplied professional expertise to populations who had little access to professional care."[38] When Haileybury was largely destroyed by fire in 1922, Laura "was on the first emergency train" to reach the town.[39] Her pioneering work laid the foundations for an enormously successful Red Cross outpost system in Ontario.[40]

In 1923 she became the director of the Welfare Division of the Public Health Department of Toronto.[41] In 1927 she moved to Vancouver, where she revolutionized the Children's Aid Society and guided three new pieces of legislation to fruition: the Infants Act, the Adoption Act, and the Children of Unmarried Parents Act.[42] Throughout the 1930s and 1940s, she was instrumental in transforming child welfare in British Columbia. Her positions included Superintendent of Neglected Children and Deputy Superintendent of Child Welfare, and she ended her career as the first woman adviser to the Minister of Health and Welfare.[43] Throughout her time in BC, she was "involved in almost everything of policy significance in health and welfare and social services throughout the province."[44] She also lectured in both the nursing and social welfare programs at the University of British Columbia. In 1934, Holland was awarded the CBE for her "work in organising and developing outpost welfare services and child protection work in Eastern and Western Canada,"[45] and in 1950, an honorary doctorate from UBC for her lifetime achievements. The changes she wrought in Ontario and BC resonated throughout the twentieth century. Undoubtedly, her war experiences shaped her choice of postwar occupation; as her letters demonstrate, interacting with child refugees in Salonika had made her thoughtful about their place and education in the postwar world. Three decades later, during the Second World War, she noted in an article for *Canadian Welfare* that "war conditions (and there is reason to believe post-war conditions also) present many problems that threaten child life and suggest the need to be on the alert to devise and support measures for the protection of normal family life."[46] Her incisive study concluded with a sentence that recalls John McCrae's First World War poem "In Flanders Fields": "to Councils ... we hand the torch, with faith that they will continue to hold aloft the light for the children of today, and prepare a better world for the children of tomorrow."

Laura's mother, to whom she had written her long, detailed wartime letters, moved with her to Vancouver. Mrs. Holland died there in 1936, much mourned by the community and her daughter's friends.[47] Laura's cousin,

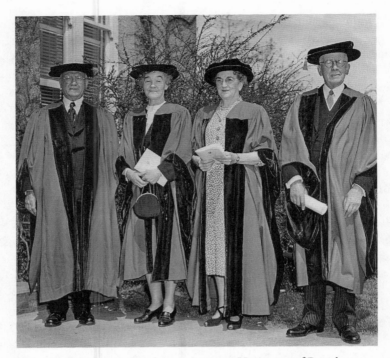

Laura Holland, honorary degree recipient, University of British Columbia, 12 May 1950. Laura is third from the left. *UBC Archives 123.1/9*

Temple Hadrill, survived his prisoner-of-war camp, married his cousin, Phyllis Hadrill, in 1920, and moved to England, where he died in 1964. Uncle George Hadrill remained as Secretary of the Montreal Board of Trade until 1924. He died in England in 1932 and was buried in Montreal.

Cairine Reay Wilson, Mildred's friend, was appointed Canada's first woman senator in 1930. She also became the first President of the League of Nations in Canada and the first Canadian female delegate to the League of Nations. She was made Chevalier de la Légion d'Honneur by the French government for her work with refugee children, and received honorary degrees from Queen's and Acadia Universities.[48] Cairine created the Mildred Hope Forbes scholarship at the MGH School for Nursing, and she kept her friend's letters throughout her lifetime.

Sarah Glassford and Amy Shaw question the "transformative effect" of the First World War on Canadian women, saying that "much-vaunted developments in labour and politics did not immediately transform either sphere."[49]

The changes that Laura and Cairine effected were broader based, affecting children, women, and families' living and working conditions through long-term health and welfare policies, thus exemplifying the "larger, longer process"[50] of women's post-war influence. Wilson's changes stemmed from her Senate position; Holland's were made more quietly. Through hard work, diplomacy, and a talent for administration, Laura Holland influenced generations of Canadians. Undoubtedly her war experiences, working with diverse populations of women and men, honed her gifts and her abilities. Other former military nurses also worked for change in diverse fields; an exploration of the postwar achievements of this group of women shows many such significant changes, albeit quietly performed.[51]

Although Laura had lost Mildred, she never forgot her wartime comrades. She joined the Canadian Overseas Nursing Association, serving as its third president from 1934 to 1936. The Association expanded individual friendships to encompass all women who had shared the experience of nursing overseas. The association became one of the first widespread professional women's organizations that was truly national in character. Its members put aside loyalties to training school and region, welcoming all nurses who had served overseas. In the postwar era, for these women, "nursing sister" was transformed from a military rank into a familial term, as the surviving nurses formed a sisterhood based on their shared wartime experiences.[52] In 1935, as president of the Canadian Overseas Nursing Association, Laura wrote to the fifteen local units, asking each to write a letter to Miss Macdonald, their former wartime matron-in-chief, telling of the unit's doings and events over the year. Margaret Macdonald was then living in Nova Scotia, struggling to start a chapter of the Overseas Nursing Association in her area.[53] "Will you join the rest of us," Laura asked, "in making Miss Macdonald's 1935 Xmas a day full of news of her over-seas family which she 'mothered' so well from 1914 to 18?"[54] The woman whom Laura had said she would "never quite forgive" was transformed into the mother of a nationwide family, someone to be cheered by her daughters' continued interest and comradeship. In this and in her other duties as president, Laura nurtured and developed the companionship and collegiality created decades earlier, when Mildred was alive and the two had shared trauma and laughter, an intense, absorbing friendship, and the shared discipline of their profession as Canadian military nurses.

Laura Holland, ARRC, CBE, LLD, died in British Columbia in 1956; her work in social welfare is still influential and remembered.

Appendix

EXCERPT FROM LAURA HOLLAND'S
1907 TRAVEL DIARY

Laura Holland was exceptionally well-travelled for her time, having grown up in Toronto, Ontario, Truro, Nova Scotia, and Montreal, Quebec, and having made trips to western Canada, England, and New York City before the war. The following diary excerpts, from her 1907 trip to New York City, show her meticulous attention to time and detail. Although her wartime diaries, or "memo-books," as she called them, have not survived, we know that she wrote brief entries daily then expanded them to create her detailed wartime letters. This trip to New York City also shows her love of adventure and her family's social status: they dined and had cocktails at the most elegant hotels, shopped at the newest department stores, hired an automobile (still rare at the time), and enjoyed both Coney Island and the Metropolitan Museum of Art.

Tuesday, August 13th, 1907

Uncle electrified us by suggesting a trip to New York ... for his holiday. Fooled round all morning ... then went downtown to ... make enquiries, which were eminently satisfactory. From there went to ball game. Toronto vs. Jersey City. Former won. Poor game, though. Mr. Roberts came to see me in the evening.

Wednesday, August 14th

Had breakfast in bed, all of us. Then I went ... & had my hair washed.... Came home in time for late lunch. Dressed & went for a walk in [High] Park after tea.

Thursday, August 15th

Hustled all morning & caught 3.45 boat to Niagara via Gorge Route. Perfect day. Arrived at 7.30, & having taken sandwiches with us, walked over to the Park, & ate them by the Rapids.

Caught 8.36 train for Buffalo, where we connected with the New York train. Pullman[1] crowded ... but as we had an upper & lower were alright.

Friday, August 16th

Very comfortable night. Arrived in Albany at 8 a.m. Went straight to wharf & caught the Hudson Day River Line boat.... Had delicious coffee & rolls on board. Such a crowd was on [but] the boat was so large & comfortable it didn't much matter. Beautiful trip down the River & we arrived at New York at 42nd St. at 7.30 p.m. Took car up to Anita's at 162 W. 46th St.[2] Found her waiting for us for dinner. After we had had a little rest ... went to Scheffle Hallë for beer.... From there took car to the "Haufbräu."[3]

Saturday, August 17th

It was quite late when we got to bed last night, so didn't get up until nearly ten. Had breakfast then took subway down to the "Aquarium." Had a good look here, then walked up Broadway. Saw Trinity Church & St. Pauls.[4] Had lunch ... then took elevated home.[5] Met Anita & went to Grand Central Station to meet Mac. He took us over to the Belmont to have a cocktail. Then we took subway away out to the Clairemont, where we had claret-cup. Had a walk along Riverside Drive, saw Grant's Monument,[6] then took just the ordinary [street]car in, which meant quite a ride. Got off at the Knickerbocker for another cocktail, & who should be at the next table having dinner but Hammerstein. From there went to the Astor House for dinner, in the "Orangery" Room, which is certainly lovely, & an awfully nice little orchestra. Had melon, Crab-a-la-Astor. Then to the Jardin de Paree, a roof-garden affair over the Criterion. From there to the Waldorf Roof-garden for drinks & dance....[7]

Sunday, August 18th

All had breakfast in bed together, Mac included. We left the house at 12.30 & took car to the Metropolitan Museum of Art, where we had a hurried glance. The Bacchante & "The Mares of Diomedes" by Borglum[8] were especially lovely. Met Mac & Anita at 3. p.m. & went straight to the Café

Martin for lunch, melon, cold meats, salad, cocktails, rhine wine cup, sweets & coffee being the order of the day. From there to the wharf, where we took the [boat] to Coney Island. Perfect day & glorious sun-set, simply beyond words. After arriving at Coney Island went into Dreamland & it is well named. They lighted up just as we arrived. The water-chute was the 1st stunt. "The Feast of Belshazzar" – rotten. Then the scenic, which was both exciting & pretty. From there walked along ... Main St. to Luna Park. Such crowds everywhere, but no wonder, for we heard afterwards there was no less than 425,000 people there. At Luna we did the Helter Skelter, Mac & Anita excepted. From there we walked to Raven Hall for dinner. Melon, Cold Lobster, salad, cocktails, beer & coffee. Then Mac brought us all home in a motor all along Coney Island Boulevard, through Brooklyn, over the new Williamsburg bridge, up through part of the Bowery, along Broadway then home —— !!!! Glorious.[9]

Monday, August 19th

Left Anita's at 8.15 supposedly to catch the 9 o'clock boat, but decided to have the day to ourselves. Took subway to the Bronx & spent the whole morning, had lunch at the Rocking Stone Restaurant. Delicious cold Lamb, salad, & coffee. Left there about three. Went & took a motor bus along Fifth Ave. When we came back went into Altman's, then Macy's.[10] Then took elevated to W. 10th St. where we went to a cunning little table D'Hote place for dinner.... Had small tables out at the back, & is run by an Italian. ... Menu. Tomatoes fixed in some weird way. Delicious pea-soup. Pigeon a-la-Bordelais, salad, Roast Beef, spaghetti, cheese (roquefort), plums & coffee. From there caught the Ferry, & went straight over to Weehawken for our train.[11] No Pullman so had to sit up all night in a crowded car, but lived through, & had many happy thoughts of New York. Train left at 8.30 p.m.

Tuesday, August 20th

Should have arrived at Buffalo at 7.30 [a.m.] but was late, & didn't get in until nearly 9 o'clock. Had breakfast in station, then took train to Niagara. Bought some lunch at the Woman's Exchange & made straight for the car as it had started to pour.... The river though looked lovely in this dull weather. Got soaking [wet] before we got on boat, but drank some whiskey & ate our lunch, then felt better. Arrived at 4 o'clock, took car home, had tea, then we spent the twilight trying to get clean, all departing for bed at nine o'clock, worn out with the effort.

Notes

Introduction

1 Mildred Forbes, letter to Mrs. Holland, June 9, 1915, University of British Columbia Archives (UBCA), Laura Holland fonds (Holland), Correspondence Series, boxes 1–2.

2 The reference to "worst station" is from Nicholson, *Canada's Nursing Sisters*, 66.

3 Letters from Laura Holland to mother, Laura Holland fonds (Holland), UBCA, Correspondence Series, boxes 1–2. Letters from Mildred Forbes (Forbes) to Cairine Wilson (Cairine), Library and Archives Canada (LAC), Cairine Reay Wilson fonds (Wilson), R5278-4-1-E, microfilm reel H-2299.

4 Laura was honoured with the military award the Associate Royal Red Cross in 1917 for her work in the Mediterranean, the Companion of the British Empire in 1934 for her work in Ontario and BC, and an honorary doctorate (LLD) by the University of British Columbia in 1950.

5 Mildred was awarded the Royal Red Cross (1st Class) in 1917. The French government awarded her the Médaille des epidémies en argent in 1919 for her work in France, and she was mentioned in despatches, a military honour, for her work as acting matron of CCS No. 2 and two Canadian Forestry Hospitals in France.

6 Cairine Wilson, born in 1885 in Montreal, was the daughter of Janet Mackay and wealthy Liberal Senator Robert Mackay. She married Norman Wilson, the MP for Russell, in 1909 and moved to Rockland, a small town about twenty miles from Ottawa. Cairine and Mildred were "close childhood friend[s]." Knowles, *First Person*, 53.

7 Interviews by the editor with Laura Holland's family member, Stephen Cooke, August 15, 2012; a colleague of Laura's, Patricia Fulton, August 17, 2012; and historian and writer Glennis Zilm, August 18, 2012.

8 For instance, in the United Kingdom, the diaries of a professional nurse, *A Nurse at the Front: The First World Diaries of Sister Edith Appleton*, ed. Ruth Cowen, and a volunteer nurse, *Dorothea's War: A First World War Nurse Tells Her Story*, ed. Richard Crewdson, are just two of the most recent British nursing narratives to be published. Since the war, nurses' narratives have been published and popular in the United Kingdom, with Bagnold, *A Diary without Dates*, and Brittain, *Testament of Youth*, being two of the best-known of the voluntary nurses' memoirs. Professional nurses' memoirs and diaries haven't been published as prolifically, but Luard's *Unknown Warriors*, one of the first to be published, has now been reprinted, as have others' works.

9 Ruby Peterkin wrote ten letters, available on LAC's virtual exhibit, *The Call to Duty*, (http://www.bac-lac.gc.ca/eng/discover/military-heritage/first-world-war/canada-nursing-sisters/

Pages/list.aspx?NurseID=102067). Luella Denton wrote twenty-one letters, available on Grey Roots Museum and Archives's virtual exhibit, *A Canadian Nursing Sister,* (http://www.greyroots.com/exhibitions/virtual-exhibits/a-canadian-nursing-sister).

10 Library and Archives Canada has posted online the narratives of six Canadian military nurses. Of these, Alice Isaacson's diary is the most sustained narrative. Isaacson was born in Ireland and trained and worked in the United States, and so does not provide the same wholly Canadian perspective as Laura and Mildred; also, Alice's diary covers only 1917 and 1918, so omits the early years of the war. The other five posted narratives, although providing valuable insights into individual experiences, are scanty and fragmentary. Dorothy Cotton's diary, written in the form of reports, and some of her letters provide a first-hand account of hospital work in Russia. Anne E. Ross, with No. 3 CSH, wrote a brief unpublished account of her war service. Laura Gamble's diary contributes a first-hand account of her experiences in Salonika, but is brief. Ruby Peterkin's letters, though fragmented, also illuminate nurses' experiences in the east, while Sophie Hoerner's letters from France provide interesting insights into the early days of the war in France. Visit *The Call to Duty: Canada's Nursing Sisters,* LAC, http://www.bac-lac.gc.ca/eng/discover/military-heritage/first-world-war/canada-nursing-sisters/Pages/canada-nursing-sisters.aspx. Similarly, Luella Euphemia Denton's twenty-one letters, housed at Grey Roots, provide a fleeting yet vital glimpse of her life on active service. Duffus published the partial diary of Elsie Dorothy Collis and photographs and records by Mary Ethel Morrison in *Battlefront Nurses of WWI.* Norris's *Sister Heroines* provides a history of Calgary nurses during the war, and includes some letters and much other valuable information. Only three nurses published memoirs in book form – Bruce, *Humour in Tragedy;* Clint, *Our Bit;* and Wilson-Simmie, *Lights Out!* – with the last two questioning, as Mann did in *The War Diary of Clare Gass* (xxv–vii), why Canadian nurses had been largely forgotten in Canadian histories of the First World War. Finally, Maude Wilkinson included her war experiences in a three-part lifetime memoir in *Canadian Nurse,* which was later expanded and published as *Four Score and Ten.* Other sources are available in archives, but are not readily available outside them.

11 Helen (Fowlds) Marryat Fonds (Marryat), Trent University Archives (TUA), 69–001, series I, box 1. Also available in *Nursing Sister Helen Fowlds: A Canadian Nurse in World War I,* http://www.trentu.ca/admin/library/archives/ffowldswelcome.htm.

12 Acton, "Writing and Waiting," 55.

13 Hanna, *Your Death Would Be Mine,* 288.

14 Roper, *The Secret Battle,* 50.

15 The artificial division of "battlefront" and "homefront" left "Canada's nurses ... in the ambiguous position of being ... an invisible group." The two visible groups were combatant soldiers and civilians living at home. Nurses – non-combatants who were part of the Canadian Army and on active service – were an anomaly. McKenzie, "'Our Common Colonial Voices,'" 94.

16 Toman, *Sister Soldiers.*

17 Nicholson, *Canada's Nursing Sisters,* 44.

18 Toman, "'A Loyal Body,'" 23. Toman's article brilliantly explores the concept of identity for these nurses.

19 Canadian nurses were granted the relative rank and the pay of lieutenants in Militia Order No. 20, January 25, 1900. Nicholson suggests that the "higher status" of the nursing profession in Canada contributed to this recognition. Nicholson, *Canada's Nursing Sisters,* 38–44, 241.

20 McPherson, *Bedside Matters*, 18.

21 Watson, *Fighting Different Wars*, 72. Watson also observes that although Nightingale revolutionized military nursing, she envisioned the work as classed, with lower-class women doing the actual work, supervised by their superiors. Watson notes: "Nightingale made nursing respectable, and then the respectable women whose employment it became took over its direction" (73). The new generation of nurses was composed mostly of middle-class women whose families could not economically support them (73–74).

22 Holland to mother, June 25, 1915; July 7, 1915.

23 Toman, "A Loyal Body," 22.

24 Mann, *The War Diary*, xxiv.

25 Toman, "A Loyal Body," 22.

26 Clint, *Our Bit*, 65. Toman also explores the fraught relations between British and Canadian nurses and authorities in "'A Loyal Body.'"

27 Allard, "Caregiving on the Front," 161–62. See also Mann, *The War Diary*, xxvii–xxvix.

28 For descriptions of war nursing work and care, see Hallett, *Containing Trauma*; Allard, "Caregiving on the Front"; and Mann, *The War Diary*. McPherson, in *Bedside Matters*, describes the six care areas that Canadian nurses had to learn during their regular three-year training program as "administrative tasks," "diagnostic testing," "assisting medical and surgical personnel," "therapeutic nursing duties" such as "counterirritants, medications," and so on, "maintenance of the ward and equipment," and "bedside care" (79–81).

29 Acton and Potter, "'These Frightful Sights,'" 61.

30 Mann, *The War Diary*, xxv. Many of the nursing sisters, including Laura and Mildred, described the strenuous work they did at Christmas to ensure a happy time for the men and the male medical staff.

31 Hanaway, "Alexander Mackenzie Forbes."

32 Alexander Casimir Galt was made KC in 1909 in Winnipeg, Manitoba, and appointed to the Court of King's Bench in 1912. Goldsborough, "Memorable Manitobans."

33 Mentioned in Laura Holland's letters as also attending the Montreal General Hospital School of Nursing, though in a different year.

34 McPherson, *Bedside Matters*, 12.

35 Holland to mother, October 30, 1915.

36 Mann comments that "Forbes's talents were exceptional, and from the time of her arrival in [Macdonald's office] in 1916, Macdonald wanted to keep her until the end of the war." Mann, *Margaret Macdonald, Imperial Daughter*, 86.

37 Laura Hadrill Holland, diaries, privately owned by Stephen Cooke.

38 Paulson, Zilm, and Warbinek, "Profile of a Leader." See also Laura's handwritten list of her positions and associated salaries. Holland fonds, UBCA, box 2.

39 Laura Holland fonds. Travel diaries, 1907, 1908, UBCA, box 2.

40 Laura signed for her graduation medal in October 1913, according to the MGH School of Nursing Registry book in the Alumnae Association Archives. However, her handwritten list of her employment lists her graduation date as 1914, the date that Paulson, Zilm, and Warbinek have used. Holland fonds, UBCA, box 2. I am grateful to Margaret Suttie of the Alumnae Association of the MGH School of Nursing for researching this information about Laura's graduation medal.

41 Canadian Forestry Corps units supplied timber and lumber for the armies. They also cleared land to construct airstrips and other sites. According to Macphail, "each of the 60 Forestry Corps Companies [in France] had small detention hospitals of 6 beds each," and there

were five additional central hospitals with larger bed capacities. Macphail, *Official History*, 223. Mildred and Laura were first posted to the hospital at Lajoux, Jura, with 150 beds, and Mildred in charge. They were then transferred to a smaller hospital in District 12, with the Bordeaux group of corps. Mildred again ran this hospital.

42 Theories of women's "autobiography" and life writing grew in tandem with the burgeoning field of women's war studies. Seminal scholars in women's autobiography include Sidonie Smith and Helen Buss. Smith, in *Subjectivity, Identity, and the Body*, posits women's writings as "resistance" to the "unified self" of maledom that marginalizes women and imposes notions of self and place upon them through a "master narrative" (17–23); Buss, in *Mapping Our Selves*, uses the metaphor of a map to convey "the ways in which humans use language to know themselves and the world" (11).

43 According to Keshen, not only were newspaper accounts censored, but authority was extended to include surveillance of telephone conversations and cables. As the war continued, the Canadian government legislated ever more elaborate and wide-reaching control and surveillance. Keshen, *Propaganda and Censorship*, 65–67.

44 Laura did consider applying for transport duty with Mildred. Eventually she decided not to, on the grounds of her mother's anxiety and her own tendency towards seasickness. Holland to mother, May 8, 1917.

45 McKenzie, "Our Common Colonial Voices, 97.

46 Fussell, in *The Great War and Modern Memory*, argues that censorship made it difficult for soldiers to write about their experiences home, and that soldiers omitted details about danger and poor conditions to spare their families anxiety. He thus entrenched the notion of "soldier's truth" versus "civilian propaganda," which Higonnet overturned as an artificial division in "All Quiet in No Women's Land."

47 I have left the numbers on Laura's letters for scholars who are interested in studying the unpublished letters. As an example of timing, around February 11, 1916, Laura received her mother's letter No. 33, then on February 18, No. 39, and the next day, nine more letters, Nos. 30 to 38, which had been written up to two-and-a-half months previously. Package delivery was even more erratic: Laura's birthday box, mailed from Canada to Lemnos in October 1915, arrived in March 1916, after the nurses had been transferred to Salonika.

48 Bakhtin, *Speech Genres*, 93–94.

49 For an extended discussion of wartime correspondence as seen through Bakhtin's theory of dialogism, see McKenzie, "Witnesses to War," or her "Correspondence, Constructs, and Qualification."

50 Both Ouditt, in *Fighting Forces, Writing Women*, 20, and Potter, in *Boys in Khaki, Girls in Print*, 189, note the religious connotations of this famous poster.

51 Holland to mother, November 23, 1915.

52 Fussell perpetuates this myth, thus creating a perceived gap of knowledge between those at home and those overseas. His assumption is not based on a thorough study of letters. Fussell, *The Great War*, 181–83. Keshen, in *Propaganda* (153–55), thoroughly explores other means of censorship in Canada but spends little time on censorship in letters and concurs with Fussell.

53 McKenzie, "Our Common Colonial Voices."

54 See Hynes, *A War Imagined*, for an extended discussion of the provisions and impact of the British Defence of the Realm Act (DORA); see Keshen, *Propaganda*, for the Canadian government's regulations.

55 British VAD nurse Vera Brittain, her QAIMNS friend Faith Moulson, and Vera's brother Edward Brittain signed the envelopes of their own letters later in the war. This honour

system bypassed the unit censor. Vera Brittain and her fiancé Roland Leighton also used codes to convey place. McKenzie, "Correspondence, Constructs, and Qualification," 260.

56 According to Helen Fowlds, Cecily Galt, Mildred's cousin and fellow nurse, was recalled to England after her father, an influential Canadian judge, raised the contents of one or more of her letters from Lemnos with the Canadian government, which in turn contacted London. Marryat, TUA, diary, November 20, 1915; letter to mother, February 18, 1916.

57 Holland to mother, January 22, 1916.

58 For an analysis of Mildred's subtle overturning of regulations, see McKenzie, "'Our Common Colonial Voices,'" 116–17.

59 Forbes to Cairine, July 27, 1917.

60 Holland to mother, November 23, 1915.

61 McKenzie, "Our Common Colonial Voices," 115.

62 McKenzie, "Witnesses to War," 26.

63 Forbes to Cairine, October 22, 1915.

64 Holland to mother, May 7, 1916.

65 Forbes to Cairine, August 27, 1917.

66 See Helen Fowlds Marryat in note 11.

67 See notes 9 to 11 for a complete listing of publicly available accounts.

68 Mann, *The War Diary*, xl.

69 Stuart, "Social Sisters," 25, 23.

70 Ibid., 23.

71 Toman, "A Loyal Body," 17.

72 See the Conclusion and Epilogue for Laura's postwar accomplishments, career, and awards.

73 Toman, "A Loyal Body," 19–20.

74 Holland to mother, February 21, 1916.

75 Toman, "A Loyal Body," 12.

76 Holland to mother, November 28, 1915; January 15, 1916; August 26, 1915.

77 Hallett's excellent *Containing Trauma*, for instance, which explores the actual wartime nursing practices of Allied military nurses, is based on a multitude of first-person accounts but includes only two Canadian military nurses, while *Veiled Warriors*, her superb history of the Allied nursing forces, only infrequently gives the Canadian nurses' perspectives. Harris expands the conception of Australian First World War nurses' work in *More Than Bombs and Bandages*, a fascinating work built on and around many Australian nurses' own words, indicating the richness of Australian resources available for such explorations. Other work done includes Watson's important distinction between the attitudes of voluntary and professional nurses towards their war service in *Fighting Different Wars*; Acton's inclusion of war nurses' trauma and grief in *Grief in Wartime*; Potter's literary study of specific nurses' memoirs in *Boys in Khaki*; Higonnet's introduction to the writings of Mary Borden and Ellen Lamotte in *Nurses at the Front*; and Das's exploration of the impact of touch on nursing attitudes and work in *Touch and Intimacy*. These are only a few of the works in a burgeoning field that rest on first-person narratives by war nurses. Scholars seldom include Canadians as part of their studies of British or Allied nursing. The same holds true for recent medical histories of the war: Harrison's *The Medical War* includes Australian but not Canadian experiences; and Carden-Coyne's *The Politics of Wounds* mentions Canadian units only twice and explores Gallipoli only from the Australian and British perspectives, although three Canadian hospitals contributed medical care.

78 Morin-Pelletier, *Briser les ailes de l'ange*.

79 Toman, *Sister Soldiers*.
80 Gibbon and Mathewson, *Three Centuries*; Nicholson, *Canada's Nursing Sisters*.
81 Bates, Dodd, and Rousseau, *On All Frontiers*; Allard, "Caregiving on the Front," 153–68.
82 Toman, "A Loyal Body"; Stuart, "Social Sisters."
83 McKenzie, "Our Common Colonial Voices."
84 Buss, *Mapping Our Selves*, 206.
85 Heilbrun, "Introduction," xv.
86 Vicinus, *Intimate Friends*, xvi.
87 Faderman, *Odd Girls and Twilight Lovers*, 11. Faderman rightly argues that all-girl colleges spread "what eventually [came] to be called lesbianism" by providing all-female enclaves and role models. However, she omits nursing as a form of higher education or profession (1–36).
88 Lee, "Sisterhood at the Front," 19.
89 McPherson, *Bedside Matters*, 19.
90 This phenomenon is similar to what Faderman claims for all-girl colleges. However, whereas for women in colleges, men "'lived' in a distant universe" (*Odd Girls*, 20), training for nurses meant contact with male doctors and patients, and war nurses were the only women in a sea of men.
91 For statistics about the numbers of overseas military nurses who married or remained working in various fields, see Morin-Pelletier, "Héritières de la grande guerre."
92 Vance, *Death So Noble*, 128.
93 Ibid.
94 Bourke, *Dismembering the Male*, 127–28.
95 Lee, "Sisterhood at the Front," 16.
96 Watson, *Fighting Different Wars*, 86.
97 Ibid.
98 Watson, "A Sister's War," 108.
99 Ibid., 105. Watson notes that TFNS Alice Slythe's diary "focused more on the novel than the familiar" and that "her professionalism all but erased both wards and warriors from her account." After reading Watson, I noted the same tendency in Laura's and Mildred's letters. At times, both struggle to write interesting letters because nothing new had happened; the work is routine and their setting has not changed.
100 Bertha Ann Merriman fonds, Ontario College of Nurses (OCN). Bertha's daughter wrote on the back of this photo that throughout her childhood, she remembered this photo sitting on her mother's dressing table.
101 Fowlds to mother, October 1, 1916. Marryat fonds, TUA.
102 Probably Ella Edna Willett, born 1892. She joined the CAMC in June 1915. Mildred Forbes signed as witness to Willett's attestation form, so Willett probably sailed for England on the same ship.
103 Wilson-Simmie, *Lights Out!*, 78.
104 Allard, "Caregiving on the Front," 164.
105 Macdonald, in Mann, *Margaret Macdonald*, 93.
106 Holland to mother, June 20, 1915.
107 Fowlds to mother, March 25, 1915. Marryat fonds, TUA.
108 Holland to mother, March 2, 1917.
109 Ibid., July 30, 1915.
110 Nicholson, *Canada's Nursing Sisters*, 66.

111 Forbes to Cairine, September 7, 1915. I have left this quotation unedited to provide an example of Mildred's original words.

112 Holland to mother, August 26, 1915. I have left this quote unedited to provide an example of Laura's words.

113 War Diaries, 3rd CSH, LAC, RG 9, Militia and Defence, series III-D-3, vol. 5033, reel T-10923, file 844, access code 90. *War Diaries of the First World War*, http://www.collectionscanada.gc.ca. Curiously, two sections of the War Diary note Matron Jaggard's death on different dates, September 24 and September 25. See also War Diaries, 1st CSH, LAC, RG 9, Militia and Defence, series III-D-3, vol. 5033, reel T-10922, file 842, access code 90, *War Diaries of the First World War*, http://www.collectionscanada.gc.ca.

114 Holland to mother, September 25, 1915.

115 Forbes to Cairine, October 22, 1915.

116 Holland to mother, October 8, 1915. Forbes to Cairine, October 22, 1915.

117 Forbes to Cairine, September 7, 1915.

118 Holland to mother, October 1, 1915.

119 Ibid., August 26, 1915.

120 Ibid., September 6, 1915.

121 Acton and Potter, "These Frightful Sights."

122 Forbes to Cairine, November 6, 1915.

123 Holland to mother, October 8, 1915.

124 Hallett, *Containing Trauma*, 27. Hallett argues that war nurses worked to return soldiers to a physically and emotionally whole state. Doing so was usually not possible on Lemnos due to shortages of food, water, and cleansing materials to sanitize and "contain" the spread of illness.

125 Forbes to Cairine, October 1, 1915.

126 Holland to mother, November 23, 1915.

127 For example, Kate Wilson-Simmie relates a humorous incident where orderlies "borrowed" the plank a nurse needed to cross the ditch from her tent to the mess hall. The nurse was clearly angry at the waste of time this caused her (*Lights Out!*, 83). At Salonika, Laura would relate requisitioning packing cases for her ward and sometimes being told to put them back (Holland to mother, March 22, 1916). "Borrowing" equipment and materials became an art form in the army.

128 Ibid., October 27, 1915.

129 Stuart, "Social Sisters," 31.

130 Fowlds to mother, September 23, 1915. Marryat fonds, TUA.

131 On April 26, 1916, Laura commented: "It's got to be rather a joke, the way a *few* consider that only those who came over with the first contingent really understand military work. Of course Mildred & I come under the head of 1st reinforcements!!"

132 About $25 in 1915 Canadian dollars.

133 Holland to mother, August 26, 1915.

134 Ibid., September 1, 1915.

135 Ibid., September 25, 1915; see also Fowlds to mother, September 23, 1915, and December 13, 1915. Marryat fonds, TUA.

136 Holland to mother, December 11, 1915.

137 Ibid.

138 Forbes to Mrs. Holland, June 9, 1915.

139 Holland to mother, July 21, 1915.

140 Ibid., August 26, 1915.

141 Moorehead, *Gallipoli*, 191.

142 Holland to mother, December 28, 1915.

143 Clint, *Our Bit*, 60; see also Fowlds's diary, November 19, 1915, and successive days, Marryat fonds, TUA; and Holland to mother, September 6, 1915.

144 Perhaps suspected of husband-hunting?

145 Holland to mother, October 1, 1915.

146 Ibid., May 1, 1916.

147 Ibid., May 2, 1916.

148 Holland to mother, October 27, 1915, November 28, 1915; Fowlds, Letter to Don (her brother), November 4, 1915, Marryat fonds, TUA. Mildred was more discreet about doings within the unit, but wrote frequently about overall mismanagement. See, for instance, her letter to Wilson of October 1, 1915. Clint, too, rails about the conditions and poor management in her memoir, *Our Bit*.

149 Holland to mother, November 28, 1915.

150 McKenzie, "Our Common Colonial Voices," 115–19.

151 Holland to mother, October 27, 1915; Forbes to Cairine, October 1, 1915, for instance.

152 Forbes to Cairine, October 1, 1915.

153 Toman, "A Loyal Body," 12.

154 McKenzie, "Our Common Colonial Voices," 121.

155 Mildred emphasized her annoyance with British authority right up to her last letter, where she notes the "silly rules & regulations made & enforced by a prim Matron who glared at us severely!" during their leave on the Riviera. Forbes to Cairine, January 25, 1919.

156 For instance, Mann claims that the "nurses displayed a female version of *esprit-de-corps*" and "loved their work" (*The War Diary*, xxi). Allard, too, states that the nurses' "isolation and sadness ... encouraged a sense of friendship, solidarity, and loyalty" ("Caregiving on the Front," 164), but she also notes tensions based on nurses' origins (165). Overall, such solidarity is not evident on Lemnos; however, individual friendships did develop under such harsh conditions. Helen Fowlds, for instance, developed her friendship with Myra Goodeve as a result of the unwavering humour and courage Goodeve showed on Lemnos.

157 Fowlds judged her fellow nurses severely before the rush of casualties in May 1915. After the rush, she commented that the "girls here are a mighty fine lot. You have to work <u>with</u> people to really know their value." Fowlds was much more tolerant of eccentricity after that experience. Letter to mother, May 9, 1915. Marryat fonds, TUA.

158 Watson observes this "deep and powerful comradeship" in women's postwar writing, as part of their way of remembering the war; for the nurses examined here, comradeship appeared in their war writing while the war was ongoing but after they had returned to England, comfort, and safety. Watson, *Fighting Different Wars*, 269.

159 Holland to mother, February 10, 1917.

160 Holland, Fowlds, and Merriman, as well as others who served on Lemnos, became members of the Canadian Overseas Nursing Association. Laura's travel diaries for the 1940s note a visit to Helen Fowlds Marryat in Ontario, when Laura was en route from Vancouver to Europe.

161 Forbes to Cairine, July 27, 1917.

162 Ibid., August 29, 1917.

163 Ibid.

164 Stuart, "Social Sisters," 34.

165 Ibid., 33.

166 Holland to mother, May 7, 1916.

167 Laura considered taking the portable organ with her when she left Salonika, but left it as a gift to the unit.

168 Unfortunately, this box was opened before it reached the unit, and only a glove survived.

169 Holland to mother, March 29, 1916.

170 Ibid.

171 Forbes to Cairine, January 3, 1918.

172 Holland to mother, October 1, 1915.

173 Ibid.

174 Ibid, January 7, 1916.

175 According to Laura, "Miss Macdonald took it into her head to spend Xmas [at Cheyne Place] & has taken Mildred with her, much to the latter's disgust." Miss Macdonald invited Laura for Christmas dinner, the "first time" the two had had the chance to get to know one another. Holland to mother, December 24, 1916; December 25, 1916.

176 Ibid., January 7, 1916.

177 Lee, "Sisterhood at the Front," 22. Faderman, in contrast, suggests that sexologists began classifying sexual "inversion" in the second half of the nineteenth century but that the concept and terminology did not seem to have become common knowledge until after the First World War. Faderman, *Odd Girls*, 40, 62–63; see also Nicholson, *Singled Out*, 50–51, 229–33.

178 McPherson, *Bedside Matters*, 16.

179 See Mann, *Margaret Macdonald*, 124–29.

180 See Stuart's study of Helen Fowlds in "Social Sisters," 25–39; and Ridout, *Nursing Sister*.

181 Holland to mother, September 14, 1916.

182 Forbes to Cairine, June 20, 1917.

183 Holland to mother, February 19, 1916.

184 Their younger companion, Helen Fowlds, did buy silk underwear in Cairo, but had her faded uniforms dyed back to their original colour, a much cheaper option than buying new ones in silk. Fowlds to mother, February 13, 1916. Marryat fonds, TUA.

185 Holland to mother, August 17, 1916.

186 Vance, *Death So Noble*, 10.

187 Bourke, 127–28.

CHAPTER 1: JOURNEYING TO WAR

1 Lifeboat drill. The *Lusitania* had been sunk by a German U-boat less than a month earlier with great loss of life.

2 A remedy for seasickness greatly in vogue during the war. Laura suffered from seasickness whenever she set foot on a ship.

3 Acting Matron Mildred Forbes had to call the commands for the nurses during drill.

4 Lollie and Mildred went to theatres and concerts constantly whenever they were in London, and Lollie reviewed almost every one for her mother; it was a shared interest, though space does not permit printing her reviews.

5 Matron-in-Chief Margaret Clothilde Macdonald. Born in 1873 in Nova Scotia, Macdonald trained at the New York City Hospital and nursed in the Spanish-American War, the Boer War, and Panama before becoming matron-in-chief of the CAMC nurses in August 1914. Mann, *Margaret Macdonald*.

6 When Laura and her mother visited England in 1908 or 1909, work on the Victoria Memorial outside Buckingham Palace, designed by Sir Aston Webb, was under way. The statue was unveiled in May 1911.

7 "Clivedon," the nickname for the Duchess of Connaught's Canadian Red Cross Hospital on the Astor's estate of Cliveden at Taplow. Laura misspells the estate name as "Clivedon" throughout her letters.

8 So called because they were selected to join Canadian General Hospital No. 3, organized by McGill University in 1915.

9 Charlotte Christina Jack, born 1889.

10 Dorothy Cotton, a graduate of the Royal Victoria Hospital in Montreal, had an unusual war; she was sent to Russia to represent Canada and did two tours of duty there, experiencing the Russian Revolution in Petrograd in 1917. See her writing and photographs in "The Call to Duty: Canada's Nursing Sisters," LAC, http://www.bac-lac.gc.ca/eng/discover/military-heritage/first-world-war/canada-nursing-sisters/Pages/dorothy-cotton.aspx.

11 Martha Allan's Attestation Paper has "non-graduate nurse" under "Profession."

12 The son of Uncle George's friend, a Mr. Temple occasionally mentioned in Laura's letters.

13 Conscription began in Britain in 1916.

14 Lt.-Col. Charles William Farran Gorrell, born 1871 in Ontario, a physician and surgeon from Ottawa who was with the First Canadian Contingent. "The Duchess of Connaught Canadian Red Cross Hospital," *British Journal of Nursing*, April 17, 1915, 320.

15 Ibid. Matron Edith Campbell, born 1871, from Montreal. She was with the First Canadian Contingent.

16 The hospital was under quarantine because of a case of scarlet fever. Holland to mother, July 25, 1915.

17 Ethel Frances Upton, a trained nurse from Montreal, born 1884. Went with CSH No. 1 to Lemnos and Salonika. Cecily Galt, a cousin of Mildred Forbes, born 1888 in Toronto; a member of the influential Galt family.

18 CSH No. 1, organized in Valcartier, Quebec, in September 1914. CSH No. 1 had been posted in England and Wimereux, France, before moving to Lemnos. Stationary hospitals were designed to take in up to four hundred patients by 1915; general hospitals were larger, taking in up to 1,020 patients by 1915. Macphail, *Official History*, 214–16.

19 Eleanor Margaret Charleson, born 1878, Matron of CSH No. 1, from Ottawa, went overseas with the First Canadian Contingent in 1914; Colonel Samuel Hanford McKee, born 1874, joined CSH No. 1 when it was organized at Valcartier, Quebec, in 1914. Commanding Officer (OC) of CSH No. 1 on Lemnos until he was invalided to England.

20 No Canadian troops fought in the Dardanelles.

21 Alexandria, Egypt, a major harbour and transit centre for the Mediterranean forces.

22 CSH No. 1 had been posted to Wimereux, France, since February 1915. In July, the unit was preparing to move to Abbeville, also in France, when it was suddenly transferred to Lemnos. War Diary, CSH No. 1, July 1915.

CHAPTER 2: LEMNOS

1 Hart, *The Great War*, 168–69.

2 Moorehead, *Gallipoli*, 33.

3 The Newfoundland Regiment would join these forces in September 1915. Nicholson, *The Fighting Newfoundlander*, 163.

4 Australian and New Zealand Army Corps.

5 For a concise account of the landings and battles and an assessment of the campaign, see Hart, *The Great War*, 167–86; for an in-depth account of the conditions and the rationale of the War Council and of Sir Ian Hamilton, the Commander-in-Chief, see Moorehead, *Gallipoli*.

6 Harrison, *The Medical War*, 172, 203.

7 Moorehead, *Gallipoli*, 189.

8 Ibid., 37–38.

9 Shallow barges.

10 Black ships were "transport vessels hastily fitted out with some hospital facilities and equipment but lacking white hospital livery." Because they were not marked as hospital ships, they were prone to attack. Harris, *More Than Bombs*, Kindle location 1546–47. See also Hallett, *Veiled Warriors*, 127–28; and Harrison, *The Medical War*, 176.

11 Rees, *The Other ANZACS*, 38.

12 See Harris, *More Than Bombs*, Kindle location 1546–14, for a superb description of conditions on board the hospital ships and the nurses' responses. See also Rees, *The Other ANZACS*.

13 Moorehead, *Gallipoli*, 189. By September, up to eight hundred dysentery cases per day were being evacuated from the peninsula. Harrison, *The Medical War*, 195.

14 Ibid.

15 Nicholson, *Canada's Nursing Sisters*, 65–68.

16 Female nurses arrived to serve with Australian General Hospital No. 3 on Lemnos in August 1915, and suffered the same privations as their Canadian colleagues, if not worse. See Hallett, *Veiled Warriors*, 135–39; and Harris, *More Than Bombs*.

17 War Diary, CSH No. 1, August 22–31, 1915.

18 The Allies launched the Sari Bair offensive (August 6–21, 1915) in an attempt to break out of the tenuous beachheads and capture the ridge that ran down the centre of the peninsula. Moorehead, *Gallipoli*, 201.

19 War Diary, CSH No. 1, August 22–31, 1915.

20 Ibid., September 1915.

21 Nicholson, *Canada's Nursing Sisters*, 272–73.

22 War Diary, CSH No. 1, December 1, 1915.

23 Hart, *The Great War*, 185.

24 Macphail, *Official History*, 216.

25 No firm figures are available for the total number of patients treated during the five months on Lemnos. Unusually, CSH No. 1's War Diary does not summarize the exact intake and evacuation numbers of patients. Instead, the diary states the number of patients in hospital, usually weekly, along with the conditions treated.

26 Forbes to Cairine, October 1, 1915.

27 I have left this sentence unedited as an example of how Laura wrote when she was upset.

28 A turn-down collar instead of a high-necked one.

29 Temple Hadrill was deciding whether or not to volunteer.

30 Vermin, including fleas and lice, were rampant on Lemnos.

31 102° F = 38.9° C; 90° F = 32° C.

32 Lavatory, which would have been an outhouse.

33 Canadian military nurses wore the stars of rank on their uniforms. As the only female officers in the Allied armies, they were objects of curiosity. See Nicholson, *Canada's Nursing Sisters*; and Mann, "Introduction," in *The War Diary*.

34 Commander-in-chief of the Mediterranean Expeditionary Force.

35 Lice.

36 Rockland, where Cairine Wilson lived, was a town of about 4,000 on the Ottawa River, about twenty miles from Ottawa. Knowles, *First Person*, 51.

37 Laura had visited Winnipeg, Manitoba, on her trip west in 1907–8.

38 Diarrhea.

39 Colonel Henry Raymond Casgrain, born in Sandwich, Ontario, in 1857, OC of CSH No. 3, was indeed invalided to England. Matron Jessie B. Jaggard, born in Nova Scotia in 1873, married to Herbert A. Jaggard, died on September 24 or 25, 1915. Nursing Sister Munro died on September 8, 1915. Laura did not tell her mother at the time. War Diaries, CSH No. 3, LAC.

40 Approximately $25 in 1915 Canadian dollars.

41 Ironically, Laura and Mildred had not seen active service either, though many of the rest of their unit had.

42 An unskilled labourer.

43 Lt.-Col. E.J. Williams took over as OC after Colonel McKee was invalided back to England. Macphail, *Official History*, 216.

44 A chapter of the Imperial Order Daughters of the Empire.

45 St. Andrews-by-the-Sea in New Brunswick, where Clibrig, the Mackay family's summer residence, was located. Knowles, *First Person*, 43.

46 Shirley McKee, married to Colonel McKee, OC of CSH No. 1; Alice F. Casgrain, married to Colonel Henry Casgrain, OC of CSH No. 3. Neither was a trained graduate nurse; Mrs. Casgrain listed her occupation as "wife" on her attestation form. Both joined the CAMC as nursing sisters as a means of joining their husbands. Mrs. McKee was a friend of Laura's.

47 Male medical officers had a batman apiece and so could obtain hot water for washing. The twenty-six nurses had two batmen for the entire unit and so they had to wash in cold.

48 The *Gazette* (Montreal) and the *Montreal Star*, both large daily newspapers.

49 Goodwin's of Montreal, a major department store on St. Catherine Street.

50 Laura's letters were censored, and she was not supposed to give out military information. Her comment was buried deep inside a twenty-eight-page letter.

51 Stationary hospitals' bed capacity in 1915 was supposed to be four hundred. Macphail, *Official History*, 216.

52 Small barges or boats.

53 Mildred's birthday.

54 An elegant hotel, the height of luxury for the day.

55 Laura's birthday.

56 About 50 cents per pound in 1915 Canadian dollars. The price of a pound of good-quality biscuits in Canada was 15 cents, according to the *Eaton's Fall/Winter Catalogue*.

57 Kitchener inspected the troops on Lemnos at this time. According to Mabel Clint's account, he didn't enter the hospital's huts. Clint, *Our Bit*, 76.

58 Probably Cecily Galt, Mildred's cousin, daughter of Alexander Casimir Galt, a judge in Winnipeg, Manitoba and a member of the politically influential Galt clan. She was sent back to England, but according to Helen Fowlds, refused to retract her story about conditions. She continued to nurse throughout the war and was awarded the ARRC. Fowlds, letter to Mother, February 27, 1916. Marryat fonds, TUA.

59 Wool blankets made by the famous Jaeger company.

60 It froze, snowed, and stormed.

61 Laura kept a memo book similar to the travel diary included in the Appendix. She included dates, times, and an account of the money she spent. The wartime memo books have not survived.

62 Matron Charleson, accompanied by Nursing Sister Florence Hunter, left for Alexandria on December 8, 1915. According to Hunter's diary, the two had Christmas dinner at the Hotel Majestic with friends and attended a dance. They set sail for Lemnos on December 27. Florence Hunter Ridout, Diary, December 8–27, 1915, Canadian War Museum, 58A 1 235.1, 20070103–002.

63 One of the first brands of instant coffee.

64 Boned, stuffed turkey.

65 A popular brand of camera.

Chapter 3: Alexandria and Cairo

1 A luxury hotel built beside the Nile in Cairo.

2 The Canadian nurses were under British regulations during their stay.

3 Canadian nurses, as officers, were allowed to go out on expeditions with officers, usually in pairs, but were not permitted to go out with the men.

4 The Mena House Hotel. Laura wrote her letter home on its notepaper.

5 Out of uniform.

6 Rebecca Hervey, born 1874.

7 Probably Margaret Jane Kingston, born 1883. She joined the CAMC on May 27, 1915.

8 Laura probably meant the Mosque of Muhammed Ali Pasha, or the Alabaster Mosque.

9 This letter exemplifies the "diary letters" that Laura wrote whenever she was travelling on leave.

10 Mabel Clint survived her phlebitis, was invalided back to Canada, and fought her way back overseas to France later in the war. War Service Record.

Chapter 4: Salonika

1 Mazower, *Salonica*, 275–76. In the Second Balkan War in 1913, Bulgaria attempted to take over Salonika but was defeated by Greece (278–79).

2 Venizelos was forced to resign, though he was restored to power later in the war. Hart, *The Great War*, 187–88.

3 Mazower, *Salonica*, 284.

4 Hart, *The Great War*, 189.

5 Later in the war, as many as 400,000 troops were stationed in the area of Salonika. Harrison, *The Medical War*, 231.

6 Mazower, *Salonica*, 289. Venizelos set up a "provisional government" in Salonika in 1916, in direct opposition to King Constantine in Athens. Constantine was forced into exile in 1917 (286–88).

7 Nicholson, *Canada's Nursing Sisters*, 72–73.

8 Hart, *The Great War*, 194–95.

9 Ibid., 195.

10 Holland to mother, March 11, 1916.

11 Harrison, *The Medical War*, 233.

12 War Diary, CSH No. 1, June to August 1916.

13 Ibid., July 1, 1916. Matron Charleson was invalided to England on July 1.

14 Frances Athill Harman, born in Toronto in 1881, had served at Dr. Depage's *L'ambulence de l'océan* in Belgium. She joined the CAMC at the beginning of October 1915 and travelled to Lemnos to join CSH No. 1 as a reinforcement.

15 In fact, Laura and Mildred became good friends in Salonika with Helen Fowlds and Myra Goodeve, who were fond of fun and very social. They would visit Helen whenever possible when all were back in England.

16 A main street in Montreal.

17 This comment confirms that Cairine and Mildred went to the same school, "Misses Symmers and Smith" in Montreal. Knowles, *First Person*, 38.

18 Anzac Cove, one of the Gallipoli landing beaches.

19 Laura's birthday was on November 14, so this box probably would have been packed and shipped in early or mid-October.

20 Though the sector was relatively quiet for infantry, Salonika was subject to air raids.

21 The camp had a Zeppelin air raid on March 27 at 5 a.m. Helen Fowlds wrote in her diary, "The costumes were varied and original. Drysdale had a pair of pyjamas tucked into the tops of her stockings – her boots, laces untied and dragging, and British warms. Ida with curlers and her long uniform coat. Mae went around mostly in a wonderful lingerie nightie, pink bed jacket etc. ... Forbes and Holland were in red, rather peevish at being wakened so early." Diary, Marryat fonds, TUA, March 27, 1916.

22 Mildred also hints at the air raids.

23 Also known as Lake Koroneia, about 8 kilometres from present-day Thessaloniki.

24 Forward observation posts were dug out in front of the first line of trenches in no man's land to allow closer scrutiny of the enemy's movements.

25 A telling comment. Laura was used to china.

26 CGH No. 4 (University of Toronto) was organized in March 1915. It served at Salonika from November 1915 to May 1916, then moved to Kalamaria, about 7 kilometres from Salonika, where it remained until August 1917, then returned to England. CGH No. 5 was organized in Victoria, BC, in May 1915, and posted to Salonika from December 1915 to August 1917, when it returned to England. Macphail, *Official History*, 214–17.

27 CSH No. 3 did indeed go to France, but CSH No. 5 became CGH No. 7 in January 1916 and remained in Cairo. Macphail, *Official History*, 214–17.

28 According to Bertha Merriman, shortly after CSH No. 1 arrived in Salonika, a suggestion was made that the nurses and medical officers share the same mess – in essence, eat together. The nurses objected strongly. Letter to father, March 15, 1916, Merriman fonds, AOnt.

29 The nurses had had a special trench dug for them for air raids.

30 Georgianna ("Georgie") McCullough, born in Ottawa in 1887, joined the CAMC in September 1914 and travelled overseas with the First Canadian Contingent.

31 Catherine Scoble, born in 1886, joined the CAMC in September 1914 and went overseas with the First Canadian Contingent.

32 About 42°C.

33 From 35 to 42°C.

34 40 to 41°C.

35 A bacterial or fungal infection of the abdomen caused by a rupture, puncture, or medical complication of another condition. "Peritonitis," *Mayo Clinic*, www.mayoclinic.org.

36 Florence Hunter. See Ridout, ed. *Nursing Sister Florence Alexandria Hunter.*

37 A bacterial or staphylococcus infection that usually needs to be opened to drain, as Mildred's was. Treatment included applying hot, moist cloths to the infected area.

38 A balance scale with counterweights.

39 Diarrhea.

40 A type of horse-drawn carriage.

CHAPTER 5: ENGLAND

1 Further air raids would occur until August 1918, causing the British government to impose blackout regulations on potential target areas. Castle, *London*, 60–63; see also Kennett, *The First Air War*.

2 Macphail, *Official History*, 145–69.

3 Due to space limitations, I have cut many of Laura's letters home for this period. Her almost daily recounting of the two's activities shows that Laura fitted visits to her many relatives into odd hours off when Mildred was working. Full days off were always spent together, as were teatimes and any other times the two could arrange. Their social life was full and busy. Because Mildred met most nurses returning from overseas postings at the office, Laura and Mildred enjoyed many teas, dinners, and theatre performances with their fellow nurses.

4 Matron-in-Chief Macdonald's office. All nurses reported in when they returned from abroad.

5 Laura repeatedly told her mother that she was well throughout her time in Salonika, but for about three weeks, her letters were surprisingly short. She put that down to the heat, but it's entirely possible that she was ill. However, most of the nurses returning from the Mediterranean were debilitated and given at least five weeks of medical leave.

6 While abroad, CAMC nurses were required to wear uniform on- and off-duty. In 1914 and 1915, they were also required to do so in England, but that requirement was changed.

7 Laura and Mildred each bought a suit, Laura's of dark blue cloth with a hairline stripe. She delighted in nice clothing, though she disliked the amount of time that shopping took.

8 Germany began Zeppelin bombing raids on England in 1915, but the raid on September 2, 1916, was the largest of the war. Sixteen airships attacked London on this date. Castle, *London*, 60.

9 Laura would have been granted free room and board in the hospital.

10 While in London, Laura reverted to diary letters, where she recounted the pair's doings almost daily.

11 In Salonika, CSH No. 1 cared for over four hundred patients with twenty-six nurses, some of whom would have been on night duty and some off sick. Having eight nurses care for twenty-six patients meant a high level of individual care.

12 Lady Julia Drummond, an influential philanthropist from Montreal, headed the Red Cross Information Bureau in London during the war. "Mrs. George A. Drummond, Lady Drummond," McCord Museum, Montreal. http://www.mccord-museum.qc.ca.

13 Laura probably meant December 26, since her letter is about December 25.

14 General Jones was then head of the CAMC at HQ.

15 Laura's original sentence began with "It would mean" and continued to the end of this paragraph, a sure sign that she was agitated.

16 The distinctive medium-blue uniform the nurses wore on the wards, as opposed to their dark-blue dress uniform.

17 The throne room.
18 At least one page is missing from the letter at this point.
19 The Canadians launched a large trench raid on February 28 in the Vimy sector. Two waves of gas were released towards the German lines, but the Germans, protected by respirators, swept the attackers with concentrated fire. Many wounded Canadians died of gas poisoning when the second wave rolled back towards the Canadian lines. Cook, *Shock Troops*, 61–71.
20 Telegrams, or "cables," were the fastest way to contact those at home or overseas. News of service personnel who were injured, died of wounds or illness, or killed in action was delivered by cable to relatives' homes. By 1917, just receiving a telegram could be a shock.
21 Laura had a number of relatives in England on both sides of her family. She and Mildred were visiting Nancy Budgett.
22 As Mildred was to find out, CCS No. 2 was subjected to shelling and air raids and was eventually shelled out. War Diary, CCS No. 2; see also Mann, *The War Diary*.
23 A small hospital for officers only near Tunbridge Wells in East Sussex. Macphail, *Official History*, 222.
24 This letter is the last one extant written by Laura to her mother.

CHAPTER 6: FRANCE

1 This photo, titled "A Canadian Casualty Clearing Station 'Somewhere in France,'" was published in *Canada* in December 1917. Mildred mentions it in her letter of February 12, 1918, as one of the photos taken of CCS No. 2 in the summer of 1917. *Canada*, December 29, 1917, 387.
2 War Diary, Second Canadian Casualty Clearing Station (CCS No. 2), July 14, 1917.
3 For instance, on August 5, a bomb fell fifty yards from the nurses' quarters. War Diary, CCS No. 2.
4 For a vivid description of work at a CCS and its impact on an individual nurse, see Wilson-Simmie, *Lights Out!*, 143–50; and Clare Gass's diary entries from November 2, 1917, to June 29, 1918, in Mann, *The War Diary*, 178–97.
5 War Diary, CCS No. 2, July 14, 1917.
6 Hart, *The Great War*, 351.
7 *Regulations*, https://archive.org/details/regulationsforcaoocanauoft.
8 These casualties occurred during the Battle of the Menin Road Bridge on September 20.
9 War Diary, CCS No. 2, September 30, 1917.
10 The Battle of Poelcapelle on October 9 and the First Battle of Passchendaele on October 12.
11 War Diary, CCS No. 2, October 31, 1917.
12 Hart, *The Great War*, 364.
13 These figures are calculated from the War Diary, CCS No. 2, for this time period.
14 Interestingly, CCS No. 2's War Diary reports that Matron E. Ridley inspected the CCS on March 13, and a concert was given that same day. Laura and Mildred left for fourteen days' leave on March 13, returning on March 27. War Diary, CCS No. 2, March 13–29, 1917.
15 War Diary, CCS No. 2, August 22, 1918; see also Forbes to Cairine, August 21, 1918.
16 The Canadians' unofficial name for this operation was Llandovery Castle, "in homage" to the Canadian hospital ship that was torpedoed and sunk in June 1918; fourteen nurses died, some known to Mildred and Laura. Cook, *Shock Troops*, 417.

17 War Diary, Canadian Forestry Corps, District 12, LAC, RG 9 III-D-3, vol. 5017, states that a new hospital was constructed at Facture in early October; given the places Mildred names in her letters, it is most likely this hospital that the two were posted to.

18 Censorship was very heavy at CCSs. Mildred and Laura could not tell their relatives where they were or about the actions taking place in Flanders.

19 CGH No. 3 (McGill) was organized in Montreal in March 1915, served in England until June 1915, and was then posted to France (Dannes-Camier until January 1916, then Boulogne), where it remained until 1919. The nurses for the unit were selected from the two main English-speaking nursing schools, the Montreal General and the Royal Victoria. Fetherstonhaugh, *No. 3 Canadian*.

20 Many convoys arrived at night.

21 Harriet Graham, born in 1883 in Nova Scotia. Nursing Sister Graham was awarded the RRC in 1917.

22 The Third Battle of Ypres.

23 The War Diary records heavy bombardments, enemy airships circling overhead, and casualties from shelling or bombing at nearby CCSs throughout July and August.

24 Cairine's husband, Norman Wilson, was the manager of W.C. Edwards and Company's lumber mills, built on the Ottawa river in Rockland. Knowles, *First Person*, 49.

25 Robert Moyse, born 1889, lived on Sherbrooke Street in Montreal.

26 Ethel Boultbee, from Vancouver, had served with Mildred and Laura on Lemnos and in Salonika.

27 The Canadians had taken the village of Passchendaele earlier in November; British and Australian troops had tried, only to fail.

28 Major Henry Willis-O'Connor.

29 Probably Lt.-Gen. Arthur Currie, in charge of the Canadian forces.

30 Probably Lt. Edward Baldwin Savage of Montreal.

31 Lt.-Col. Wilfrid Bovey and Major Edward Phillips Fetherstonhaugh.

32 Third son of Queen Victoria and governor general of Canada from 1911 to 1916.

33 Most likely nearby Bailleul, but possibly Boulogne.

34 Rhoda Blanche Wurtele, born 1883, joined the CAMC in Ottawa in 1916.

35 Mildred's brother, Kenneth Forbes.

36 War Diary, CCS No. 2, April 14 to 30, 1918. See also Mann, *The War Diary*, 193–94.

37 Vermin.

38 Mary Lucretia Domville, born 1881 in New Brunswick, but with family in Montreal. Edith Wilson was probably a relative of Cairine's husband.

39 Hope Wurtele Macdougall. Mildred was related to the Galts and knew the Tuppers.

40 Dunkirk, about 25 kilometres from Esquelbecq, was on the coast.

41 A hint that the course of the war and its advances and retreats affected the CCS and its facilities.

42 St. Omer, about 30 kilometres from Esquelbecq, was a transfer point to reach Calais or Boulogne.

43 Fourteen Canadian military nurses died when a German U-boat sank the hospital ship *Llandovery Castle* off the Irish coast on June 27, 1918. On May 19, 1918, one nurse was killed, two died of wounds, and five were injured in an air raid at CGH No. 1 at Etaples. On May 30, 1918, three nurses were killed at CSH No. 3 in Doullens in an air raid. Nicholson, *Canada's Nursing Sisters*, 92–97.

44 Cairine Wilson's older sister, Anna Loring, who was in Britain during the war and also corresponded with Mildred.
45 Lucy Gertrude Squire, born 1884.
46 In early October, the Austrian and German governments began suing for peace as the result of Allied advances.
47 Rhoda Wurtele, a nursing sister who had been at CCS No. 2, became a friend of Mildred's. Her sister obviously was not.
48 Cairine's oldest brother Angus died in June 1918, and if her new baby was a boy, would take his name.
49 The Rockland lumber mills were sold in 1918, and Norman Wilson formed a new partnership with four others in an Ottawa lumber operation. Knowles, *First Person*, 58.
50 Mildred's older half-brother, Dr. Alexander Mackenzie Forbes.
51 In southwestern France.
52 This epidemic became global, killing more people than had died in the war.
53 The war ended on November 11, 1918.
54 Anna Margaret, born December 9, 1918. Knowles, *First Person*, 58.
55 Mildred's sister's child, Mildred Hope Burrill. Laura Holland would leave her a legacy in her will.

CONCLUSION AND EPILOGUE

 1 Mann, "Where Have All the Bluebirds Gone?," 36.
 2 Acton and Potter, "These Frightful Sights," 4.
 3 Ibid.
 4 Ouditt, "Tommy's Sisters," 739. Found in Potter, *Boys in Khaki*, 153.
 5 Potter, *Boys in Khaki*, 153.
 6 Holmes, "Day Mothers and Night Sisters," 44.
 7 Acton, *Grief in Wartime*, 3.
 8 Holland to mother, September 6, 1915.
 9 Forbes to Cairine, September 7, 1915.
10 Ibid.
11 Holland to mother, August 26, 1915; Forbes to Cairine, October 1, 1915.
12 Holland to mother, October 1, 1915.
13 Ibid., October 1, 1915
14 McKenzie, "'Our Common Colonial Voices,'" 115–17.
15 Ibid.; Holland to mother, October 30, 1915.
16 Toman, "A Loyal Body," 17.
17 War Diary, CCS No. 2.
18 Forbes to Cairine, August 28, 1917.
19 Ibid.
20 Ibid.
21 Holland to mother, August 25, 1915.
22 Ibid., November 28, 1915.
23 Ibid.
24 Ibid., March 11, 1916.
25 Ibid., November 4, 1915; Forbes to Cairine, November 6, 1915.
26 Holland to mother, February 24, 1917; March 2, 1917.

27 Ibid., March 4, 1917.
28 Vance, *Death So Noble*, 128.
29 Forbes to Cairine, October 31, 1918.
30 *The Microcosm 1920*, Simmons College Annual, vol. II (Boston: Students of Simmons College), 140.
31 *Canadian Nurse* 17.2 (February 1921), 99.
32 *Public Health Journal* 12.6 (June 1921), 277. See also Morin-Pelletier, "A la fois infirmière."
33 *Canadian Nurse* 17.2 (February 1921), 99.
34 *The Gazette* (Montreal), January 13, 1921, 7.
35 *Public Health Journal* 12.6 (June 1921), 277.
36 *Canadian Nurse* 19.1 (January 1923), 41.
37 Wilkinson, *Four Score and Ten*. Wilkinson, another war veteran, succeeded Laura Holland at the Red Cross, and her memoir mentions the two working together as Laura helped Wilkinson understand the work.
38 Dodd, Elliott, and Rousseau, "Outpost Nursing in Canada," 139.
39 Paulson, Zilm, and Warbinek, n.p.
40 For a description of the beginnings and rise of Ontario Red Cross outposts, see Elliott, "'Keep the Flag Flying.'" Elliott mentions that many records were destroyed shortly before she began her research; perhaps this destruction is the reason why Laura Holland is rarely mentioned in histories of the Ontario Red Cross outpost hospitals. Her successor, Maude Wilkinson, also a former First World War military nurse, recounts Laura training her for the work and assuring Maude that "there never seemed to be any conflict" with the Outpost Hospital Committee. "'They asked for her opinion,' Miss Holland commented, 'and usually accepted it.'" Wilkinson, *Four Score and Ten*, 95.
41 *Canadian Nurse* 19.7 (July 1923), 422.
42 Paulson, Zilm, and Warbinek, n.p.
43 Ibid.
44 Ibid.
45 Laura Holland, CBE citation card, *London Gazette*; citation and award privately owned by Stephen Cooke.
46 Holland, "A Better World," 9.
47 Laura Holland fonds, UBCA.
48 LAC, "Cairine Reay Wilson, Biography."
49 Glassford and Shaw, "Introduction," 20.
50 Ibid.
51 See Morin-Pelletier, "Héritières," for the postwar work that many overseas nurses performed in diverse fields.
52 Emmeline Robinson, Scrapbook of the Edmonton Unit, Canadian Association of Registered Nurses of Alberta Archives (CARNA). Robinson included a picture of a tree in the scrapbook, with small photographs of the nurses in their uniforms pasted to the branches.
53 As late as 1937, Miss Macdonald was still struggling to start a branch of the Overseas Nursing Association in her part of Nova Scotia. In 1937, she succeeded in getting nine nurses together to mark Remembrance Day. Letter from Margaret Macdonald to Mrs. Taylor, Edmonton Unit, December 6, 1937, in Robinson, Scrapbook of the Edmonton Unit, 1920–1945, CARNA. The Edmonton Unit sent her greetings every year at Christmas and other holidays.
54 Letter from Laura Holland to Mrs. Harold Orr, President, Edmonton Unit, Canadian Overseas Nursing Association, November 4, 1935. In Robinson, Scrapbook, CARNA.

APPENDIX

1 A car with berths for overnight travellers.
2 Between 6th and 7th Avenues in midtown.
3 German beer garden restaurant.
4 Still standing at Wall Street and Broadway.
5 Rapid transit railways that ran above the city streets.
6 Tomb of President Ulysses S. Grant.
7 A whirlwind tour of Manhattan's most elegant hotels.
8 Bronze sculpture, 1905.
9 Luna Park, a famous amusement park. The Helter Skelter was a spiral stone slide, daring for the time.
10 Two famous department stores on 34th Street.
11 Weehawken, New Jersey, a transportation hub.

Bibliography

ARCHIVAL COLLECTIONS

Alumnae Association of the Montreal General Hospital School of Nursing Archives, Montreal
Registry Book of Graduating Nurses

Archives of Ontario (AOnt)
Robert Owen and Bertha Ann Merriman fonds, MU 7809

Canadian Association of Registered Nurses of Alberta Archives and Museum (CARNA)
Scrapbook of the Edmonton Unit of the Overseas Nursing Association, 1920–1945. Compiled by Emmeline Robinson. CARNA 91.21.

Canadian War Museum (CWM)
Florence Hunter Ridout fonds. Diary and photograph albums. CWM 20070103–002.
Ethel Frances Upton fonds. Photograph album. CWM 19790413–012.
Images of No. 2 Casualty Clearing Station. CWM 19800795–002.

College of Nurses of Ontario (CNO)
Bertha Ann Merriman fonds

Grey Roots Museum and Archives (GRMA)
A Canadian Nursing Sister: Luella Euphemia Denton. http://www.greyroots.com/exhibitions/virtual-exhibits/a-canadian-nursing-sister.

Library and Archives Canada (LAC)
Mildred Forbes. Overseas experiences as nurse during the first World War, personal. Cairine Reay Wilson fonds. Letters from Mildred Hope Forbes to Cairine Wilson. R5278–4-1-E, Microfilm reel H-2299.
The Call to Duty: Canada's Nursing Sisters. LAC archived virtual exhibit. http://www.collectionscanada.gc.ca/nursing-sisters/025013-2200-e.html.
Dorothy Cotton fonds. R2677–0-3-E. Also available in *The Call to Duty*.
Laura A. Gamble fonds. R2699–0-4-E. Also available in *The Call to Duty*.
Sophie Hoerner fonds. R2495–0-7-E. Also available in *The Call to Duty*.
Alice E. Isaacson fonds. R11203–0-1-E. Also available in *The Call to Duty*.
Ruby Gordon Peterkin fonds. R7630–0-X-E. Also available in *The Call to Duty*.

Anne E. Ross fonds. R2672–0-7-E. Also available in *The Call to Duty.*

Soldiers of the Great War (CEF Database).

War Diaries, 1st Canadian Stationary Hospital. RG9, Militia and Defence, Series III-D-3, vol. 5033, reel T-10922, file 842, access code 90. *War Diaries of the First World War.* http://www.collectionscanada.gc.ca.

–, 2nd Canadian Casualty Clearing Station, RG 9, Militia and Defence, Series III-D-3, vol 5032, reel T-10921–10922, file 839, Access code 90. *War Diaries of the First World War.* http://www.collectionscanada.gc.ca.

–, 3rd Canadian Stationary Hospital. RG 9, Militia and Defence, Series III-D-3, vol. 5033, reel T-10923, file 844, access code 90. *War Diaries of the First World War.* http://www.collectionscanada.gc.ca.

War Diary, Canadian Forestry Corps, District 12 (Bordeaux Group), LAC, RG 9 III-D-3, vol. 5017.

War Service Record, Eleanor Charleson, RG 150, accession 1992–93/166, box 1643–21.

–, Mildred Forbes, RG 150, accession 1992–93/166, box 3183–3.

–, Cecily Galt, RG 150, accession 1992–93/166, box 3388–13.

–, Laura Holland, RG 150, accession 1992–93/166, box 4441–1.

–, Bertha Merriman, RG 150, accession 1992–93/166, box 6131–44.

–, Helen Fowlds, RG 150, Accession 1992–93/166, box 839–62.

McGill University Archives
Montreal General Hospital School of Nursing Archives, RG 96

Trent University Archives (TUA)
Helen Marryat fonds (Marryat), 69–001, series I, box 1. Also in *Nursing Sister Helen Fowlds: A Canadian Nurse in World War I.* http://www.trentu.ca/admin/library/archives/ffowldswelcome.htm.

University of British Columbia Archives (UBCA)
Laura Holland fonds (Holland), Correspondence Series; Diary Series; Miscellaneous and Memorabilia Series, Photographs, boxes 1–2. Also UBC Historical Photograph Database, 123.1.

Private Collections
Laura Hadrill Holland, Diary, 1876, 1879, 1886. Formerly owned by Stephen D. Cooke. Now at the McCord Museum, Montreal.

Photographs and family documents.

NEWSPAPERS AND PERIODICALS

Canada. An Illustrated Weekly Journal for All Those Interested in the Dominion. London, Montreal.

The Canadian Nurse; The Canadian Nurse and Hospital Review. Vancouver: Canadian National Association of Trained Nurses.

Public Health Journal [Canadian Journal of Public Health]. Toronto: Canadian Public Health Association.

The Gazette (Montreal).

The London Gazette.

The Microcosm. Simmons College Annual. Boston, MA.

OTHER SOURCES

Acton, Carol. *Grief in Wartime: Private Pain, Public Grief.* New York: Palgrave Macmillan, 2007. http://dx.doi.org/10.1057/9780230801431

–. "Writing and Waiting: The First World War Correspondence between Vera Brittain and Roland Leighton." *Gender and History* 11, 1 (1999): 54–83. http://dx.doi.org/10.1111/1468-0424.00129

Acton, Carol, and Jane Potter. "'These Frightful Sights Would Work Havoc with One's Brain': Subjective Experience, Trauma, and Resilience in First World War Writings by Medical Personnel." *Literature and Medicine* 30, 1 (Spring 2012): 61–85. http://dx.doi.org/10.1353/lm.2012.0010

Allard, Geneviève. "Caregiving on the Front: The Experience of Canadian Military Nurses during World War I." In *On All Frontiers: Four Centuries of Canadian Nursing,* ed. Christina Bates, Dianne Dodd, and Nicole Rousseau, 153–67. Ottawa: University of Ottawa Press, 2005.

Appleton, Edith. *A Nurse at the Front: The First World Diaries of Sister Edith Appleton.* Ed. Ruth Cowen. London: Simon and Schuster, 2012.

Bagnold, Enid. *A Diary without Dates.* 1918. Fairfield, UK: Echo Library, 2014.

Bakhtin, Mikhail. *Speech Genres and Other Late Essays.* Trans. Vern W. McGee. Austin: University of Texas Press, 1986.

Bassett, Jan. *Guns and Brooches: Australian Army Nursing from the Boer War to the Gulf War.* Melbourne: Oxford University Press Australia, 1992.

Bates, Christina, Dianne Dodd, and Nicole Rousseau, eds. *On All Frontiers: Four Centuries of Canadian Nursing.* Ottawa: University of Ottawa Press, 2005.

Bourke, Joanna. *Dismembering the Male: Men's Bodies, Britain, and the Great War.* Chicago: University of Chicago Press, 1996.

Brittain, Vera. *Testament of Youth: An Autobiographical Study of the Years 1900–1925.* London: Virago, 2004 [1933].

Bruce, Constance. *Humour in Tragedy: Hospital Life behind Three Fronts.* London: Skeffington, 1918?.

Buss, Helen M. *Mapping Our Selves: Canadian Women's Autobiography in English.* Montreal and Kingston: McGill-Queen's University Press, 1993.

"A Canadian Casualty Clearing Station 'Somewhere in France.'" (Photograph of CCS No. 2, Remy Siding, France). *Canada,* December 29, 1917, 387.

Carden-Coyne, Ana. *The Politics of Wounds: Military Patients and Medical Power in the First World War.* Oxford: Oxford University Press, 2014.

Castle, Ian. *London, 1914–17: The Zeppelin Menace.* Oxford: Osprey Publishing, 2008.

Clint, Mabel. *Our Bit: Memories of War Service by a Canadian Nursing-Sister.* Montreal: Alumnae Association of the Royal Victoria Hospital, 1934.

Cook, Tim. *Shock Troops: Canadians Fighting the Great War, 1917–1918 .* Vol. 2. Toronto: Viking, 2008.

Crewdson, Dorothea. *Dorothea's War: A First World War Nurse Tells Her Story.* Ed. Richard Crewdson. London: Phoenix, 2013.

Das, Santanu. *Touch and Intimacy in First World War Literature.* Cambridge: Cambridge University Press, 2005.

Dodd, Dianne, Jayne Elliott, and Nicole Rousseau. "Outpost Nursing in Canada." In *On All Frontiers: Four Centuries of Canadian Nursing,* ed. Christina Bates, Dianne Dodd, and Nicole Rousseau, 139–52. Ottawa: University of Ottawa Press, 2005.

Duffus, Maureen. *Battlefront Nurses of WWI*. Victoria: Town and Gown Press, 2009.

Elliott, Jayne. "Keep the Flag Flying": Medical Outposts and the Red Cross in Northern Ontario, 1922–1984. PhD diss., Queen's University, 2004.

Faderman, Lillian. *Odd Girls and Twilight Lovers: A History of Lesbian Life in Twentieth-Century America*. New York: Penguin, 1992.

Fetherstonhaugh, R.C. *No. 3 Canadian General Hospital (McGill), 1914–1919*. Montreal: Gazette Printing, 1928.

Fussell, Paul. *The Great War and Modern Memory*. London: Oxford University Press, 1975.

Gibbon, John Murray, and Mary S. Mathewson. *Three Centuries of Canadian Nursing*. Toronto: Macmillan, 1947.

Glassford, Sarah, and Amy Shaw. "Introduction: Transformation in a Time of War?" In *A Sisterhood of Suffering and Service: Women and Girls of Canada and Newfoundland during the First World War*, ed. Sarah Glassford and Amy Shaw, 1–23. Vancouver: UBC Press, 2012.

Goldsborough, Gordon. "Memorable Manitobans: Alexander Casimir Galt." *Memorable Manitobans*. Manitoba Historical Society. www.mhs.mb.ca.

Hallett, Christine. *Containing Trauma: Nursing Work in the First World War*. Manchester: Manchester University Press, 2009.

–. *Veiled Warriors: Allied Nurses of the First World War*. Oxford: Oxford University Press, 2014.

Hanaway, Joseph. "Alexander Mackenzie Forbes." *Dictionary of Canadian Biography*. http://www.biographi.ca/en/bio/forbes_alexander_mackenzie_torrance_15E.html

Hanna, Martha. *Your Death Would Be Mine: Paul and Marie Pireaud in the Great War*. Cambridge, MA: Harvard University Press, 2009.

Harris, Kirsty. *More Than Bombs and Bandages: Australian Army Nurses at Work in World War I*. Newport, Australia: Big Sky Publishing, 2011. Kindle edition.

Harrison, Mark. *The Medical War: British Military Medicine in the First World War*. Oxford: Oxford University Press, 2010. http://dx.doi.org/10.1093/acprof:oso/9780199575824.001.0001

Hart, Peter. *Gallipoli*. Oxford: Oxford University Press, 2011. Kindle edition.

–. *The Great War: A Combat History of the First World War*. Oxford: Oxford University Press, 2013.

Heilbrun, Carolyn G. "Introduction." In Vera Brittain, *Testament of Friendship*, xv–xxxii. N.p.: Wideview Books, 1981.

Higonnet, Margaret. "All Quiet in No Women's Land." In *Gendering War Talk*, ed. Miriam Cooke and Angela Woollacott, 205–26. Princeton: Princeton University Press, 1993.

–. *Nurses at the Front: Writing the Wounds of the Great War*. Boston: Northeastern University Press, 2001.

Holland, Laura. "A Better World for the Children of Tomorrow." *Canadian Welfare* 19, 8 (March 1944).

Holmes, Katie. "Day Mothers and Night Sisters: World War I Nurses and Sexuality." In *Gender and War: Australians at War in the Twentieth Century*, ed. Joy Damousi and Marilyn Lake, 43–59. Cambridge: Cambridge University Press, 1995.

Hynes, Samuel. *A War Imagined: The First World War and English Culture*. London: The Bodley Head, 1990.

Kennett, Lee. *The First Air War, 1914–1918*. New York: Macmillan, 1991.

Keshen, Jeffrey A. *Propaganda and Censorship during Canada's Great War*. Edmonton: University of Alberta Press, 1996.

Knowles, Valerie. *First Person: A Biography of Cairine Wilson, Canada's First Woman Senator*. Toronto: Dundurn Press, 1988.

Lee, Janet. "Sisterhood at the Front: Friendship, Comradeship, and the Feminine Appropriation of Military Heroism among World War I First Aid Nursing Yeomanry (FANY)." *Women's Studies International Forum* 31, 1 (2008): 16–29. http://dx.doi.org/10.1016/j.wsif.2007.11.005

Luard, Kate. *Unknown Warriors*. London: Chatto and Windus, 1930. Reprinted as *Unknown Warriors: The Letters of Kate Luard, RRC and Bar, Nursing Sister in France, 1914–1918*. Port Stroud, UK: History Press, 2014.

Macphail, Sir Andrew. *Official History of the Canadian Forces in the Great War, 1914–19: The Medical Services*. Ottawa: F.A. Acland, 1925.

Mann, Susan. *Margaret Macdonald, Imperial Daughter*. Montreal and Kingston: McGill-Queen's University Press, 2005.

–, ed. *The War Diary of Clare Gass, 1915–1918*. Montreal and Kingston: McGill-Queen's University Press, 2000.

–. "Where Have All the Bluebirds Gone? On the Trail of Canada's Military Nurses, 1914–1918." *Atlantis* 26, 11 (2001): 35–43.

Mazower, Mark. *Salonica, City of Ghosts: Christians, Muslims, and Jews, 1430–1950*. New York: Vintage Books, 2004.

McKenzie, Andrea. "Correspondence, Constructs, and Qualification in World War I." *Canadian Journal of Communication* 26, 2 (2001): 255–75.

–. "'Our Common Colonial Voices': Canadian Nurses, Patient Relations, and Nation on Lemnos." In *Other Fronts, Other Wars? First World War Studies on the Eve of the Centennial*, ed. Joachim Bürgschwentner, Matthias Egger, and Gunda Barth-Scalmani, 92–124. Leiden: Brill, 2014.

–. "Witnesses to War: Discourse and Community in the Letters of Vera Brittain, Roland Leighton, Edward Brittain, Geoffrey Thurlow, and Victor Richardson, 1914–1918." PhD diss., University of Waterloo, 2000.

McPherson, Kathryn. *Bedside Matters: The Transformation of Canadian Nursing, 1900–1990*. Toronto: University of Toronto Press, 2003.

Moorehead, Alan. *Gallipoli*. Ware: Wordsworth Editions, 1997.

Morin-Pelletier, Mélanie. "A la fois infirmière et travailleuse sociale: Les infirmières militaires et le service sociale en santé dans l'entre-deux-guerres." In *L'incontournable caste des femmes: Histoire des services de santé au Québec et au Canada*, ed. Marie-Claude Thifault, 185–204. Ottawa: Les Presses de l'Université d'Ottawa, 2012.

–. *Briser les ailes de l'ange: Les infirmières militaires canadiennes (1914–1918)*. Montreal: Athéna éditions, 2006.

–. "Héritières de la grande guerre: Les infirmières militaires Canadiennes durant l'entre-deux-guerres." PhD diss., Université de Ottawa, 2010.

"Mrs. George A. Drummond, Lady Drummond." *McCord Museum*, Montreal. www.mccord-museum.qc.ca/en/

Nicholson, G.W.L. *Canada's Nursing Sisters*. Toronto: A.M. Hakkert, 1975.

–. *The Fighting Newfoundlander: A History of the Royal Newfoundland Regiment*. Montreal and Kingston: McGill-Queen's University Press, 2006.

Nicholson, Virginia. *Singled Out: How Two Million Women Survived without Men after the First World War*. London: Penguin, 2008.

Norris, Marjorie. *Sister Heroines: The Roseate Glow of Wartime Nursing*. Calgary: Bunker to Bunker Publishing, 2002.

Ouditt, Sharon. *Fighting Forces, Writing Women: Identity and Ideology in the First World War*. London: Routledge, 1990.

—. "Tommy's Sisters: The Representation of Working Women." In *Facing Armageddon: The First World War Experienced*, ed. Hugh Cecil and Peter H. Liddle, 736–51. London: Cooper, 1996.

Paulson, Esther, Glennis Zilm, and Ethel Warbinek. "Profile of a Leader: Pioneer Government Advisor Laura Holland." *Nursing Leadership* online 13, 3 (2000).

"Peritonitis." *Mayo Clinic*, http://www.mayoclinic.org

Potter, Jane. *Boys in Khaki, Girls in Print*. Oxford: Oxford University Press, 2005.

Regulations for the Canadian Medical Service, 1914. Ottawa: Government Printing Bureau, 1915. https://archive.org/details/regulationsforca00canauoft

Rees, Peter. *The Other ANZACS: Nurses at War, 1914–18*. Crows Nest: Allen and Unwin, 2008.

Ridout, Peter H., ed. *Nursing Sister Florence Alexandria Hunter [Ridout]: The Experiences of a Nursing Sister during the Great War*. Peter H.H. Ridout, 2006.

Roper, Michael. *The Secret Battle: Emotional Survival in the Great War*. Manchester: Manchester University Press, 2010.

"Sir Samuel Hughes." *Canadian War Museum*. www.warmuseum.ca

Smith, Sidonie. *Subjectivity, Identity, and the Body: Women's Autobiographical Practices in the Twentieth Century*. Bloomington: Indiana University Press, 1993.

Stuart, Meryn. "Social Sisters: A Feminist Analysis of the Discourses of Canadian Military Nurse Helen Fowlds, 1915–18." In *Place and Practice in Canadian Nursing History*, ed. Jayne Elliott, Meryn Stuart, and Cynthia Toman, 25–39. Vancouver: UBC Press, 2008.

Toman, Cynthia. "'A Loyal Body of Empire Citizens': Military Nurses and Identity at Lemnos and Salonika, 1915–17." In *Place and Practice in Canadian Nursing*, ed. Jayne Elliott, Meryn Stuart, and Cynthia Toman, 8–24. Vancouver: UBC Press, 2008.

—. *Sister Soldiers of the Great War: The Nurses of the Canadian Army Medical Corps*. Vancouver: UBC Press, 2016.

Vance, Jonathan. *Death So Noble: Memory, Meaning, and the First World War*. Vancouver: UBC Press, 1997.

Vicinus, Martha. *Intimate Friends: Women Who Loved Women, 1778–1928*. Chicago: University of Chicago Press, 2006.

Watson, Janet S.K. "A Sister's War: The Diaries of Alice Slythe." In *First World War Nursing: New Perspectives*, ed. Alison S. Fell and Christine E. Hallett, 103–20. New York: Routledge, 2013.

—. *Fighting Different Wars: Experience, Memory, and the First World War in Britain*. Cambridge: Cambridge University Press, 2004.

Wilkinson, Maude. *Four Score and Ten: Memoirs of a Canadian Nurse*. Brampton: Margaret Armstrong, 2003.

Wilson-Simmie, Katherine. *Lights Out! The Memoir of Nursing Sister Kate Wilson, Canadian Army Medical Corps, 1915–1917*. Ottawa: CEF Books, 2004.

Index

Note: "(i)" after a page number indicates an illustration.